Molecular Modelling of Vitamin B$_{12}$ and Its Analogues

Molecular Modelling of Vitamin B$_{12}$ and Its Analogues

Penny Poomani Govender
Francis Opoku
Olaide Olalekan Wahab
Ephraim Muriithi Kiarii

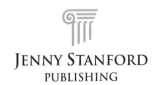

Published by

Jenny Stanford Publishing Pte. Ltd.
Level 34, Centennial Tower
3 Temasek Avenue
Singapore 039190

Email: editorial@jennystanford.com
Web: www.jennystanford.com

British Library Cataloguing-in-Publication Data
A catalogue record for this book is available from the British Library.

Molecular Modelling of Vitamin B_{12} and Its Analogues

Copyright © 2022 by Jenny Stanford Publishing Pte. Ltd.
All rights reserved. This book, or parts thereof, may not be reproduced in any form or by any means, electronic or mechanical, including photocopying, recording or any information storage and retrieval system now known or to be invented, without written permission from the publisher.

For photocopying of material in this volume, please pay a copying fee through the Copyright Clearance Center, Inc., 222 Rosewood Drive, Danvers, MA 01923, USA. In this case permission to photocopy is not required from the publisher.

ISBN 978-981-4877-58-9 (Hardcover)
ISBN 978-1-003-21339-0 (eBook)

Contents

Preface	xi

1. Introduction — 1
    1.1   Background — 1
    1.2   Causes of Vitamin B_{12} Deficiency — 2
    1.3   Uses and Effectiveness — 3
    1.4   Side Effects and Safety — 3
    1.5   Functions of Vitamin B_{12} — 4
    1.6   Exercises — 5

2. Structure, Constitution and Properties of Vitamin B_{12} — 9
    2.1   Vitamin B_{12} Structure — 9
    2.2   Main Properties of Vitamin B_{12} — 12
    2.3   Exercises — 12

3. Nomenclature — 15

4. B_{12} Organometallic Reactivity — 21
    4.1   Introduction — 21
    4.2   Cobaloxime Model Systems — 24
        4.2.1   Formation of CoX Bonds — 24
        4.2.2   Cleavage of Co–C Bonds — 25
        4.2.3   Electrochemistry — 26
        4.2.4   Alkene Coupling — 28
        4.2.5   Ring Expansion Reactions — 29
    4.3   Computational Studies on Organometallic Chemistry — 30

5. Coenzyme B_{12}–Dependent Enzymes — 39
    5.1   Introduction — 39
    5.2   Methylcobalamin — 42
        5.2.1   Methionine Synthase — 42
        5.2.2   Methylated-thiol-Coenzyme M Methyltransferase — 43
    5.3   Adenosylcobalamin — 44

vi | Contents

5.4	Hydroxocobalamin		44
5.5	Cobamamide		45
5.6	Cyanocobalamin		46

6. Recent Trends ... **51**

6.1	Introduction		51
6.2	Vitamin B_{12} for Cyanide Detection and Detoxification		52
6.3	Vitamin B_{12} for Diagnosis and Therapy		53
	6.3.1	Diabetes Mellitus	53
	6.3.2	Cardiovascular Disease	54
	6.3.3	Epilepsy	55
	6.3.4	Cancer	56
	6.3.5	Dementia	56
	6.3.6	Renal Disease	57
6.4	Antivitamins B_{12}		59
6.5	Vitamin B_{12} in Biological Systems		62

7. Catalysis ... **73**

7.1	Introduction		73
7.2	Concept of Catalysis		74
7.3	Types of Catalysis		75
	7.3.1	Homogenous Catalysis	75
	7.3.2	Heterogeneous Catalysis	75
7.4	Vitamin B_{12}: A Unique Natural Organometallic Catalyst		77
7.5	Catalytic Features of Cobalamins		80
	7.5.1	Availability	80
	7.5.2	Balance between Stability and Reactivity	80
	7.5.3	Recoverability	81
	7.5.4	High Activity-to-Dosage Ratio	81
7.6	Chemistry of the Organometallic Co–C Bond in Vitamin B_{12} Derivatives		81
7.7	Factors Controlling the Co–C Bond Cleavage		83
	7.7.1	Positional Influence of Neighbouring Ligands	83
		7.7.1.1 Trans influence of the alpha axial ligand	84

| | | 7.7.1.2 | Cis influence of the equatorial ligand | 85 |

	7.7.2	Nature of the Alpha Axial Ligand	85
	7.7.3	Presence of an Enzyme	85
		7.7.3.1 Caging effect	86
		7.7.3.2 Distortion effect	86
		7.7.3.3 Mutual stabilisation between the Co^{2+} state and the enzyme	86
7.8	Exercises		87

8. Vitamin B$_{12}$–Catalysed Reactions — **91**

8.1	Introduction		91
8.2	Vitamin B_{12} Enzymes and Their Functions		92
	8.2.1	B_{12}-Binding and B_{12}-Transporting Proteins	92
	8.2.2	Methyltransferases	92
	8.2.3	Cobalamin-Dependent Enzymes	93
8.3	Cobalamin-Mediated Organic Reactions		93
	8.3.1	Rearrangement (Isomerisation)	94
	8.3.2	Methyl Transfer Reaction (Transmethylation)	95
	8.3.3	Dehalogenation	97
	8.3.4	C–C and C–X Multiple Bond Hydrogenation	100
	8.3.5	1,4-Addition to Double Bonds	103
		8.3.5.1 Scheffold principles of cobalamin-mediated 1,4-addition reactions	104
	8.3.6	Ring-Opening Reactions	105
	8.3.7	Coupling Reactions	106
		8.3.7.1 Halide coupling reaction of alkyl halides (Scheme 8.7a)	107
		8.3.7.2 Alkene coupling reaction of styrene derivatives (Scheme 8.7b)	108
	8.3.8	Cyclopropanation	109
	8.3.9	Oxidation	111
	8.3.10	Ring Expansion Reactions	113
8.4	Exercises		113

9. Vitamin B$_{12}$ Derivatives — 117

9.1	Vitamin B$_{12}$ as an Active Ingredient of Supplements	120
9.2	Efficacy Spectrum of Bioactive Vitamin B$_{12}$ Forms	120
	9.2.1 Cyanocobalamin vs. Hydroxocobalamin	120
	9.2.2 Cyanocobalamin vs. Methylcobalamin	121
	9.2.3 Exercises	121
9.3	Methylcobalamin	122
	9.3.1 Mechanisms Underlying the Analgesic Action of MeCbl	123
	9.3.1.1 Enhancing the nerve conduction velocity	123
	9.3.1.2 Improving the rejuvenation of wounded nerves	124
	9.3.1.3 Constraining ectopic spontaneous release	124
	9.3.2 Exercises	124
9.4	Adenosylcobalamin	124
	9.4.1 Exercises	129
9.5	Cyanocobalamin	129
	9.5.1 Chemical Reactions	130
	9.5.2 Exercises	131
9.6	Hydroxocobalamin	131
	9.6.1 Special Effects of Hydroxocobalamin	131
	9.6.1.1 Long-lasting effects and sustained release	131
	9.6.1.2 Detoxing and quitting smoking	132
	9.6.1.3 Blocking nitrosative stress	132
	9.6.1.4 Hydroxocobalamin supplements: pills and capsules	132
	9.6.2 Exercises	132

10. Theoretical Approach — 139

10.1	Mechanism of the S_1 Excited-State Internal Conversion in Vitamin B$_{12}$	139
10.2	Influence of the α (Axial)–Ligand	141

10.3	Electronic and Steric Effects	142
10.4	Bond Dissociation Energies	147
	10.4.1 Exercises	149
10.5	Structural and Electronic Properties of Vitamin B_{12}	150

Index 159

Preface

For many years, the chemistry of vitamin B_{12} and its derivatives has been investigated for their inherent eco-friendly and nontoxic nature. This vitamin, also known as cobalamin, is an organic complex that contains a cobalt ion in its structure. Its derivatives are vital bio-inorganic cofactors and possess complex and rich photolytic properties, facilitated by their excited states. However, studies on vitamin B_{12} derivatives are still ongoing, with huge possibilities still available. Due to the size and complexity limitations associated with vitamin B_{12} derivatives, the main technique for investigating the ground-state properties is density functional theory (DFT). An analysis of the electronic excitation is essential to offer a detailed understanding of the photochemical reactions of vitamin B_{12} derivatives. Normally, time-dependent DFT (TD-DFT) is the best approach that can be employed to evaluate the excited states of vitamin B_{12}. Several investigations in the field of organic chemistry have effectively applied vitamin B_{12} as a catalyst in several organic reactions, such as 1,4-additions to activated double bonds, alkyl and aryl halide dimerization, dehalogenation and hydrogenation of double bonds. The capability of vitamin B_{12} to catalyse these thermodynamically challenging reactions has captured attention for future research, which can lead to revolutionary catalytic innovations. The potential energy surface associated with the excited states of vitamin B_{12} provides the most reliable approach to analyse the photophysical and photochemical properties. This book highlights the application of vitamin B_{12} as an environmentally benign catalyst for several organic reactions. It discusses the recent advances and the current understanding of the photolytic properties of vitamin B_{12} derivatives from the perspective of the density functional theory. We hope that anyone involved in nanotechnology, macromolecular science, cancer, and drug-delivery research will find this book useful.

Penny Poomani Govender
Francis Opoku
Olaide Olalekan Wahab
Ephraim Muriithi Kiarii
April 2021

Chapter 1

Introduction

1.1 Background

The long-term effects of poor nutrition which continues over generations are of much worry globally [1]. Vitamin B_{12} is only prepared by microorganisms in nature and, hence, is obtained by human beings via their diet [2]. Vitamin B_{12} (cobalamin), the only naturally biomolecule with a carbon–metal bond, is among the most vital molecules in medicine and food [3]. Vitamin B_{12} a complex water-soluble organic compounds within a tetrapyrrole ring containing Co as a central atom, which is vital to several animals and microorganisms, including humans [3]. Active forms of vitamin B_{12} are commercially available: adenosylcobalamin, cyanocobalamin and methylcobalamin. Vitamin B_{12} aids in the formation of red blood cells and the normal functioning of the nervous system and the brain. Vitamin B_{12} plays a vital role in neurologic function, growth of the myelin sheath and normal DNA synthesis [3, 4]. Vitamin B_{12} is also an essential micronutrient significant for cardiovascular, cognitive and hemopoietic functions [5]. Animal foods, such as dairy products, fish, liver and meat (e.g. yoghurt, cheese and milk), are the main dietary sources of vitamin B_{12}. It is also present in cobalamin-synthesising oysters and bacteria. Nonetheless, vitamin B_{12} is not present in plants [6]. Several studies disapprove with these findings

---

Molecular Modelling of Vitamin B_{12} and Its Analogues
Penny Poomani Govender, Francis Opoku, Olaide Olalekan Wahab, and Ephraim Muriithi Kiarii
Copyright © 2022 Jenny Stanford Publishing Pte. Ltd.
ISBN 978-981-4877-58-9 (Hardcover), 978-1-003-21339-0 (eBook)
www.jennystanford.com

Introduction

[7], but new reports have revealed that plant cells have the capability to produce comparable vitamin B_{12} compounds which participate with vitamin B_{12} for the same cellular receptors [8].

1.2 Causes of Vitamin B_{12} Deficiency

Vitamin B_{12} deficiency is a usual diagnosis, particularly in older persons [9]. Frequently the deficiency is because of mutations in the genes encoding vital proteins in the diet (vegetarian), cobalamin metabolism and reduced production of stomach acids, which are required for vitamin B_{12} absorption [10]. Traditionally, vitamin B_{12} deficiency is caused by a low concentration of vitamin B_{12} in the plasma or serum of the patient [11]. These findings are disapproved by several studies which claim that an important proportion of persons with a high or normal concentration of vitamin B_{12} normally have a deficiency [12]. The risk for vitamin B_{12} deficiency is higher with increasing age and varies with gender. Vitamin B_{12} deficiency is particularly common in older persons because of the intrinsic factor and a lack of malabsorption [13]. Vitamin B_{12} in fortified bread and milk is about 55%–60% absorbed by persons over 60 years [14]. Malabsorption from food, insufficient intake and other medical conditions are causes of vitamin B_{12} deficiency [15]. Nonetheless, human body storage of vitamin B_{12} is high, and it is broadly present in food. An earlier report reveals that low folate, high serum homocysteine and low vitamin B_{12} concentration can be related to dementia, cognitive decline and poor cognitive function [16]. Normal serum vitamin B_{12} concentrations range from 200 to 900 pg/ml, where serum levels of <200 pg/ml suggest deficiency and concentrations of <100 pg/ml typically induce neurologic damage or megaloblastic anaemia [17]. Vitamin B_{12} deficiency induces neurologic damage, megaloblastic anaemia and gastrointestinal lesions [13]. Neurologic symptoms include neuropsychiatric disorders [18, 19], mood changes without anaemia, weakness, memory loss, ataxia and paresthesias [20]. Vitamin B_{12} deficiency may also result in nerve degeneration, cardiovascular disease, pernicious anaemia because of the failure of red blood cell formation, weight loss, constipation, nausea, weakness, irreversible neurological damage and fatigue because of the failure to repair the myelin sheath protecting the nerve cells [4, 21, 22]. Pernicious anaemia is a disease characterised by the impaired production of red blood cells. Neurologic sequelae as a result of vitamin B_{12} deficiency comprise demyelination of the corticospinal tract and dorsal columns, peripheral neuropathy and paresthesias. The long-term effects of vitamin B_{12} deficiency include adverse effects on vascular health, cognition and pregnancy [23]. Several reports have shown that low vitamin B_{12} in pregnant women is related with high blood pressure in offspring [24], low levels of high-density lipoprotein cholesterol [25] and foetal growth restriction [26]. Vitamin B_{12} supplements have been effective in reducing the risk of cardiovascular diseases [27] and improving the pregnancy outcome [28]. Thus, vitamin B_{12}–fortified foods can act as an effective approach to enhance the vitamin B_{12} levels in pregnant women, the elderly and children [29].

1.3 Uses and Effectiveness

Vitamin B_{12} can be applied to the skin either by blending with avocado oil or alone for eczema and psoriasis. Moreover, vitamin B_{12} nasal gel is used against pernicious anaemia and inhibiting other vitamin B_{12} deficiency. Also, vitamin B_{12} is taken by mouth for the immune system, mental function, Alzheimer's disease and memory loss and to slow ageing and increase concentration, energy and mood. Vitamin B_{12} is likewise used for clogged arteries, low male infertility, risk of reclogging arteries after surgery, high triglyceride levels, heart disease, skin infections, allergies, asthma, diarrhoea, mental disorders, inflammatory bowel disease, nerve damage in the feet or hands, depression, swollen tendons, schizophrenia, weak bones (osteoporosis), sleep disorders, diabetes, diabetic nerve damage and high homocysteine concentrations which can be related to heart disease.

1.4 Side Effects and Safety

Vitamin B_{12} is most possibly safe for most persons (e.g. pregnant and breastfeeding women) when applied to the skin, taken via the nose or by mouth, injected intravenously into the vein or administered as a shot. About 2.6 mcg per day of vitamin B_{12} is the permitted amount for pregnant women, while breastfeeding women should take no more than 2.8 mcg per day. Mild itching has been stated in the use of avocado oil together with vitamin B_{12} cream for psoriasis. A combination of vitamin B_6, vitamin B_{12} and folate should be avoided after receiving a coronary stent or if you are sensitive or allergic to cobalamin or cobalt. Those with Leber's disease must not take vitamin B_{12} since it can extremely damage the optical nerve and causes blindness.

1.5 Functions of Vitamin B_{12}

The main functions of vitamin B_{12} are summarised as follows [11, 30]:

- Without vitamin B_{12}, folic acid cannot be absorbed and remains trapped in the intestinal wall.
- Vitamin B_{12} takes and transports a methyl group to other molecules, such as neurotransmitters and DNA.
- It supports iron activity in the body, as well as in the synthesis of choline.
- It supports the myelin sheath around nerve structures, together with folic acid.
- It helps in the metabolism of vitamin A, particularly the absorption of carotene.
- It is involved in the synthesis of white and red blood cells, working together with folic acid.
- Vitamin B_{12} is necessary for the stability and reproduction of RNA and DNA.
- Vitamin B_{12} expedites the conversion of amino acids into neurotransmitters and hormones, together with vitamin B_6.
- It participates in the synthesis of porphyrins which are a vital component of haemoglobin.
- Vitamin B_{12} acts as a coenzyme in several enzymatic reactions.

1.6 Exercises

1. What is vitamin B_{12}?
2. How common is vitamin B_{12} deficiency?
3. Why are folic acid and vitamin B_{12} so important?
4. Name some of the causes of vitamin B_{12} deficiency.
5. What are the symptoms of vitamin B_{12} deficiency?
6. Name five foods rich in vitamin B_{12}.
7. Does the body store vitamin B_{12}?
8. Why is vitamin B_{12} important?
9. What is the chemical name of vitamin B_{12}?
10. What is the best vitamin B_{12} supplement?
11. What happens when your vitamin B_{12} is low?
12. How much vitamin B_{12} is in a glass of milk?

References

1. R. L. Bailey, K. P. West Jr, R. E. Black, The epidemiology of global micronutrient deficiencies, *Ann. Nutr. Metab.*, **66** (2015) 22–33.
2. R. Carmel, Biomarkers of cobalamin (vitamin B_{12}) status in the epidemiologic setting: a critical overview of context, applications, and performance characteristics of cobalamin, methylmalonic acid, and holotranscobalamin II, *Am. J. Clin. Nutr.*, **94** (2011) 348S–358S.
3. S. S. Kumar, R. S. Chouhan, M. S. Thakur, Trends in analysis of vitamin B_{12}, *Anal. Biochem.*, **398** (2010) 139–149.
4. S. S. Kumar, R. S. Chouhan, M. S. Thakur, Enhancement of chemiluminescence for vitamin B_{12} analysis, *Anal. Biochem.*, **388** (2009) 312–316.
5. D. Kibirige, R. Mwebaze, Vitamin B_{12} deficiency among patients with diabetes mellitus: is routine screening and supplementation justified?, *J. Diabetes Metab. Disord.*, **12** (2013) 1–6.
6. R. H. Allen, S. P. Stabler, D. G. Savage, J. Lindenbaum, Metabolic abnormalities in cobalamin (vitamin B_{12}) and folate deficiency, *FASEB J.*, **7** (1993) 1344–1353.
7. F. Watanabe, Y. Yabuta, T. Bito, F. Teng, Vitamin B_{12}-containing plant food sources for vegetarians, *Nutrients*, **6** (2014) 1861–1873.

8. M. Wolters, A. Ströhle, A. Hahn, Cobalamin: a critical vitamin in the elderly, *Prev. Med.*, **39** (2004) 1256–1266.

9. D. J. Orton, C. Naugler, S. H. Sadrzadeh, Fasting time and vitamin B_{12} levels in a community-based population, *Clin. Chim. Acta*, **458** (2016) 129–132.

10. Z. Cheng, H. Yamamoto, C. E. Bauer, Cobalamin's (vitamin B_{12}) surprising function as a photoreceptor, *Trends Biochem. Sci.*, **41** (2016) 647–650.

11. T. T. Todorova, N. Ermenlieva, G. Tsankova, Vitamin B_{12}: could it be a promising immunotherapy?, in K. Metodiev (ed.) *Immunotherapy: Myths, Reality, Ideas, Future*, InTech, Rijeka, Croatia, 2017, pp. 85–100.

12. A. Sobczyńska-Malefora, R. Gorska, M. Pelisser, P. Ruwona, B. Witchlow, D. J. Harrington, An audit of holotranscobalamin ("Active" B_{12}) and methylmalonic acid assays for the assessment of vitamin B_{12} status: application in a mixed patient population, *Clin. Biochem.*, **47** (2014) 82–86.

13. K. Okuda, Discovery of vitamin B_{12} in the liver and its absorption factor in the stomach: a historical review, *J. Gastroenterol. Hepatol.*, **14** (1999) 301–308.

14. G. K. McEvoy, American Society of Health-System Pharmacists, *AHFS Drug Information 2007*, American Society of Health-System Pharmacists, Bethesda, Md., 2007.

15. H. Stracke, A. Lindemann, K. Federlin, A benfotiamine-vitamin B combination in treatment of diabetic polyneuropathy, *Exp. Clin. Endocrinol. Diabetes*, **104** (1996) 311–316.

16. G. Li, Effect of mecobalamin on diabetic neuropathies. Beijing methycobal clinical trial collaborative group, *Zhonghua Nei Ke Za Zhi*, **38** (1999) 14–17.

17. F. Watanabe, Vitamin B_{12} sources and bioavailability, *Exp. Biol. Med.*, **232** (2007) 1266–1274.

18. G. Xu, Z.-W. Lv, Y. Feng, W.-Z. Tang, G. Xu, A single-center randomized controlled trial of local methylcobalamin injection for subacute herpetic neuralgia, *Pain Med.*, **14** (2013) 884–894.

19. G. Kaltenbach, M. Noblet-Dick, E. Andres, G. Barnier-Figue, E. Noël, T. Vogel, A.-E. Perrin, C. Martin-Hunyadi, M. Berthel, F. Kuntzmann, Réponse précoce au traitement oral par vitamine B_{12} chez des sujets âgés hypovitaminiques, in *Ann. Med. Interne*, Masson, Paris, 2003, pp. 91–95.

20. C. Ortiz-Hidalgo, George H. Whipple. Nobel Prize in Physiology or Medicine in 1934. Whipple's disease, pernicious anemia and other contributions to medicine, *Gac. Med. Mex.*, **138** (2002) 371–376.

21. M. A. Bernard, P. A. Nakonezny, T. M. Kashner, The effect of vitamin B_{12} deficiency on older veterans and its relationship to health, *J. Am. Geriatr. Soc.*, **46** (1998) 1199–1206.

22. E. C. Marley, E. Mackay, G. Young, Characterisation of vitamin B_{12} immunoaffinity columns and method development for determination of vitamin B_{12} in a range of foods, juices and pharmaceutical products using immunoaffinity clean-up and high performance liquid chromatography with UV detection, *Food Addit. Contam. Part A*, **26** (2009) 282–288.

23. F. O'Leary, S. Samman, Vitamin B_{12} in health and disease, *Nutrients*, **2** (2010) 299–316.

24. K. D. Sinclair, C. Allegrucci, R. Singh, D. S. Gardner, S. Sebastian, J. Bispham, A. Thurston, J. F. Huntley, W. D. Rees, C. A. Maloney, DNA methylation, insulin resistance, and blood pressure in offspring determined by maternal periconceptional B vitamin and methionine status, *Proc. Natl. Acad. Sci.*, **104** (2007) 19351–19356.

25. A. Adaikalakoteswari, M. Vatish, A. Lawson, C. Wood, K. Sivakumar, P. McTernan, C. Webster, N. Anderson, C. Yajnik, G. Tripathi, Low maternal vitamin B_{12} status is associated with lower cord blood HDL cholesterol in white Caucasians living in the UK, *Nutrients*, **7** (2015) 2401–2414.

26. H. Van Sande, Y. Jacquemyn, N. Karepouan, M. Ajaji, Vitamin B_{12} in pregnancy: maternal and fetal/neonatal effects – a review, *Open J. Obstet. Gynecol.*, **3** (2013) 599–602.

27. S. Sucharita, T. Thomas, B. Antony, M. Vaz, Vitamin B_{12} supplementation improves heart rate variability in healthy elderly Indian subjects, *Auton. Neurosci.*, **168** (2012) 66–71.

28. D. K. Dror, L. H. Allen, Interventions with vitamins B_6, B_{12} and C in pregnancy, *Paediatr. Perinat. Epidemiol.*, **26** (2012) 55–74.

29. L. H. Allen, How common is vitamin B_{12} deficiency?, *Am. J. Clin. Nutr.*, **89** (2009) 693S–696S.

30. M. Esperanca, *The Wonders of Vitamin B_{12}: Keep Sane and Young*, Xlibris Corporation, USA, 2011.

Chapter 2

Structure, Constitution and Properties of Vitamin B$_{12}$

2.1 Vitamin B$_{12}$ Structure

Vitamin B$_{12}$ (cobalamin), the largest molecule with a molecular weight of >1000 g, is a water-soluble vitamin [1]. The chemical structure of vitamin B$_{12}$ comprises four pyrroles in the centre of a corrin ring and a Co atom binds to (ribose)-5,6-dimethylbenzimidazole (Fig. 2.1) [2].

The cobalt can link to

- a cyanide group,
- a methyl group, as in methylcobalamin, and
- a 5'-deoxyadenosine at the 5' position, as in adenosylcobalamin (coenzyme B$_{12}$).

A specific connection to the cobalamin crystal structure has a high influence on the mechanism of the enzyme reaction. A highly toxic methylmercury ion (CH_3Hg^+) also offers an unfortunate connection with methylcobalamin. The core of the molecule is a corrin ring with several connected side substituents. The ring comprises four pyrrole subunits, bound on one side by a C–H methylene group and on opposite sides by a C–CH$_3$ methylene group and with two pyrroles bound together directly. The core of the molecule is like that of porphyrins but with one of the bridging methylene groups removed.

Molecular Modelling of Vitamin B$_{12}$ and Its Analogues
Penny Poomani Govender, Francis Opoku, Olaide Olalekan Wahab, and Ephraim Muriithi Kiarii
Copyright © 2022 Jenny Stanford Publishing Pte. Ltd.
ISBN 978-981-4877-58-9 (Hardcover), 978-1-003-21339-0 (eBook)
www.jennystanford.com

A vital feature of the corrin ring is the flexibility of the corrin system when compared to a porphyrin, where the corrin ring is less flat in the porphyrin ring. Moreover, corrin only has a conjugated chain around a part of the ring, while a porphyrin is delocalised around the entire four pyrrole rings. The central Co ion is bonded to the two ligands positioned on both α-bottom and β-upper face sides of the corrin ring and four pyrrolic N atoms. The cyanide ion is usually the fifth ligand at the β-face, while the sixth ligand below the ring is an N of 5,6-dimethylbenzimidazole. The other N is attached to a 5C sugar and bears the R5′–OH group, which, in turn, links to a phosphate group and back onto the corrin ring through one of the seven amide groups bonded to the periphery of the corrin ring.

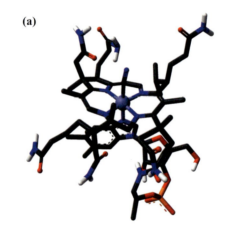

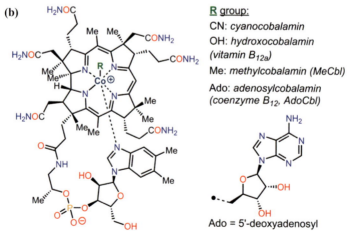

Figure 2.1 (a) 3D and (b) 2D chemical structures of vitamin B_{12} [3].

The X-ray crystal diffraction analysis of vitamin B_{12} offered the first insights into a corrin complex with a biosynthetic and structural relative to natural porphyrins [4, 5]. The corrin ligand consists of four Co-coordinating N atoms as part of a linearly π-conjugated chromophore system. Therefore, the corrin ligand is intrinsically nonplanar, and the provided coordination hole is smaller than that of the porphyrins [6]. The corrin ligand also shows a unique functionalised periphery and bound to the Co ion very strongly in natural corrinoids.

X-ray analysis was used to reveal the unique organometallic nature of coenzyme B_{12} (AdoCbl) [7]. In AdoCbl, a 5′-deoxy-5′-adenosyl group binds through a metal–C bond at the β-position of the Co ion (Fig. 2.2).

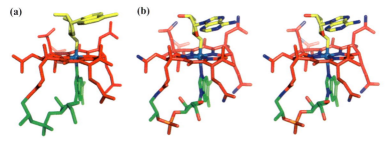

Figure 2.2 3D model of coenzyme B_{12} (AdoCbl) from X-ray analysis [7]. (a) Structure of AdoCbl in stick display style; colour representation: organometallic adenosyl group (yellow), cobalt ion (blue), nucleotide loop (green) and corrin moiety (red). (b) Stereo view of AdoCbl (hetero atoms: Co = light blue, P = yellow, O = red and N = dark blue).

X-ray analysis of cob(II)alamin (B_{12r}) revealed a pentacoordinate Co(II) centre which is similar to the Co–corrin part of the AdoCbl structure [8]. Coenzyme B_{12} structure analysis in solution via nuclear magnetic resonance (NMR) spectroscopy revealed that the organometallic 5′-deoxyadenosyl group does not bind tightly; however, it is present in two conformations around the Co–C bond [9]. The MeCbl structure was also investigated by NMR spectroscopy [10] and X-ray analysis [11], where both axial bonds of MeCbl (Co–N = 2.16 Å and Co–C = 1.98 Å) were shorter than in AdoCbl (Co–N = 2.23 Å and Co–C = 2.03 Å) [11].

2.2 Main Properties of Vitamin B_{12}

The main properties of vitamin B_{12} are as follows:

1. Vitamin B_{12} is very stable at high temperatures if the pH is between 4.5 and 5.0, whereas the strongly acidic and highly alkaline environment loses its vitamin capacity.
2. It favours proper absorption of calcium.
3. Vitamin B_{12} is negatively affected by oestrogen, sleeping pills, alcohol, etc.
4. It favours the metabolism of food (fats, carbohydrates and proteins).
5. Vitamin B_{12} is well soluble in methanol, ethanol and water.

2.3 Exercises

1. Who discovered the structure of vitamin B_{12}?
2. What is the structure of vitamin B_{12}?
3. What element does vitamin B_{12} contain?
4. What is the coenzyme of vitamin B_{12}?

References

1. B. N. Estevinho, I. Carlan, A. Blaga, F. Rocha, Soluble vitamins (vitamin B_{12} and vitamin C) microencapsulated with different biopolymers by a spray drying process, *Powder Technol.*, **289** (2016) 71–78.

2. H. Castellanos-Sinco, C. Ramos-Peñafiel, A. Santoyo-Sánchez, J. Collazo-Jaloma, C. Martínez-Murillo, E. Montaño-Figueroa, A. Sinco-Ángeles, Megaloblastic anaemia: folic acid and vitamin B_{12} metabolism, *Rev. Med. Hosp. Gen. Méx.*, **78** (2015) 135–143.

3. https://en.Wikipedia.Org/wiki/Vitamin_B12.

4. A. Eschenmoser, Vitamin B_{12}: experiments concerning the origin of its molecular structure, *Angew. Chem., Int. Ed. Engl.*, **27** (1988) 5–39.

5. M. J. Warren, E. Raux, H. L. Schubert, J. C. Escalante-Semerena, The biosynthesis of adenosylcobalamin (vitamin B_{12}), *Nat. Prod. Rep.*, **19** (2002) 390–412.

6. R. Banerjee, *Chemistry and Biochemistry of B_{12}*, John Wiley & Sons, New York, 1999.

7. D. Crowfoot-Hodgkin, Die Röntgenstrukturanalyse komplizierter Moleküle. Nobel-Vortrag am 12. Dezember 1964, *Angew. Chem.*, **77** (1965) 954–962.

8. B. Kraeutler, W. Keller, C. Kratky, Coenzyme B_{12} chemistry: the crystal and molecular structure of cob(II)alamin, *J. Am. Chem. Soc.*, **111** (1989) 8936–8938.

9. M. F. Summers, L. G. Marzilli, A. Bax, Complete proton and carbon-13 assignments of coenzyme B_{12} through the use of new two-dimensional NMR experiments, *J. Am. Chem. Soc.*, **108** (1986) 4285–4294.

10. M. Tollinger, R. Konrat, B. Kräutler, The structure of methylcob(III) alamin in aqueous solution – a water molecule as structuring element of the nucleotide loop, *Helv. Chim. Acta*, **82** (1999) 1596–1609.

11. L. Randaccio, S. Geremia, G. Nardin, J. Wuerges, X-ray structural chemistry of cobalamins, *Coord. Chem. Rev.*, **250** (2006) 1332–1350.

Chapter 3

Nomenclature

Each amide group of the five-membered pyrrolic rings are labelled from *a* to *g* and highlighted with various colours, as shown in Fig. 3.1.

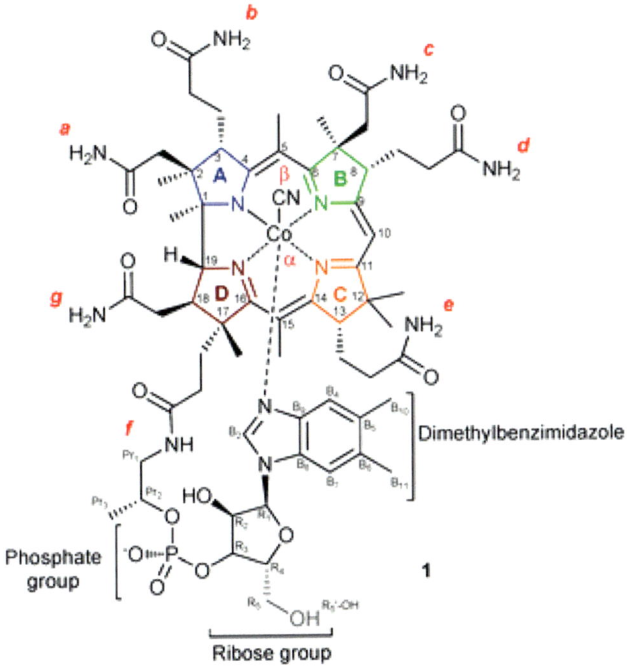

Figure 3.1 The numbering of vitamin B_{12} [1].

Molecular Modelling of Vitamin B_{12} and Its Analogues
Penny Poomani Govender, Francis Opoku, Olaide Olalekan Wahab, and Ephraim Muriithi Kiarii
Copyright © 2022 Jenny Stanford Publishing Pte. Ltd.
ISBN 978-981-4877-58-9 (Hardcover), 978-1-003-21339-0 (eBook)
www.jennystanford.com

Vitamin B_{12} (cobalamin) is a cobamide, where 5,6-dimethylbenzimidazole is bonded by a glycosyl group from its N to the C of the ribose and additionally attached by a bond between the N and the Co. The cobalamin (**1**) structure is indicated as Cbl. The term (CN) in the vitamin B_{12} abbreviation at the beginning states the presence of a cyanide ligand on the β-face side of the central Co ion. The first section of the abbreviated vitamin B_{12} name changes after changing the ligand (compounds **2–9**); for example, hydroxocobalamin is written as (OH)Cbl **2** since it has the OH ligand instead of the CN group. Anion(s) related to the corrinoids is(are) termed after the name of the (cationic) corrinoid, for example, cobamic dichloride instead of dichlorocobamic acid. The oxidation state of cobalt can be shown either after the "cob" prefix in the compound name, for example, cob(I)alamin or cob(III) alamin, or in the subscript, where vitamin B_{12s} demonstrates the +1 oxidation state, vitamin B_{12r} as the +2 oxidation state and vitamin B_{12} (compound **1**) as the +3 oxidation state. Displacement of the ribosyl-bound aglycon base from its normal coordinate bonding to position *a* of Co by another ligand (or by water) can be shown by placing the position and name of the substituting ligand before the corrinoid name and enclosing the modified corrinoid name, e.g. *Co*a-aqua-*Co*b-methyl(2-methyladenylcobamide), where the 2-methyladenyl residue is bonded to the ribose residue but is not coordinately attached to the Co atom having been displaced by water or methyl group. Methyl occupies the *Co*β position. The word "*nor*" before vitamin B_{12} indicates a lack of certain groups, for example, the methyl group at the C5, C15 or Pr_3 for compound **10**, **11** or **12** [2]. When a number is included in the vitamin B_{12} name, it signifies the position where substitution has taken place; for example, cobalamin that lacks a CH_3 group at position C5 is named as C5-*nor*-(CN)Cbl. The word "*epi*" along with the position number is used to signify a variation in the stereochemistry at that specific position, for example, 13-*epi*-derivatives which are also termed as *neo*-derivatives, as shown in Fig. 3.2.

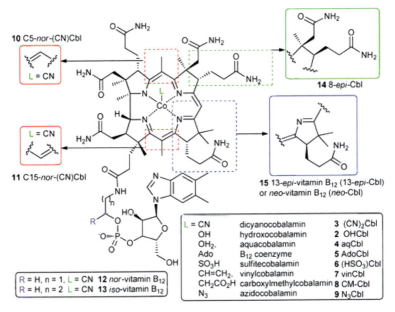

Figure 3.2 Nomenclature of vitamin B$_{12}$ [3].

Cobalamins may be termed as "cobamides" according to the following patterns, for example:

- Coa-[a-(5,6-dimethylbenzimidazolyl)]-Cob-nitritocobamide, also termed as "vitamin B$_{12c}$," is named nitritocobalamin.
- Coa-[a-(5,6-dimethylbenzimidazolyl)]-Cob-hydroxocobamide, also termed as "vitamin B$_{12b}$," is named hydroxocobalamin.
- Coa-[a-(5,6-dimethylbenzimidazolyl)]-Cob-aquacobamide, also termed as "vitamin B$_{12a}$," is named aquacobalamin, which is the conjugate acid of hydroxocobalamin.
- Coa-[a-(5,6-dimethylbenzimidazolyl)]-Cob-cyanocobamide, also termed as "vitamin B$_{12}$," is named cyanocobalamin.

Cobinamide (Cbi) **16** in Fig. 3.3 can be obtained after cleavage of the ribose moiety, in addition to the dimethylbenzimidazole and phosphate groups, which also applies to Cbi derivatives, as in (CN) Cbi, except that the central Co now has two CN groups—(CN)$_2$Cbi; see compounds **17–19**.

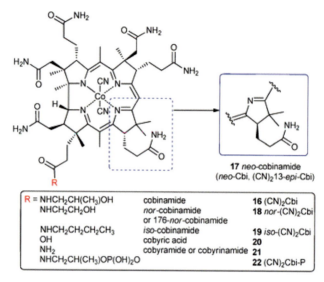

Figure 3.3 Nomenclature of cobinamide and its derivatives [3].

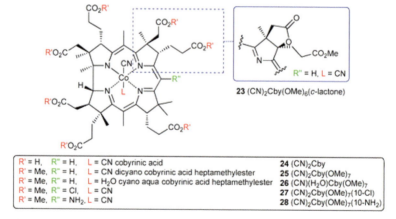

Figure 3.4 Nomenclature of cobyrinic acid and its derivatives [3].

Cobyric acid (compound **20**) can be obtained after elimination of the 2-hydroxypropyl ligand at position *f*. If position *f* bears a terminal amide (CONH$_2$) group instead of a carboxylic acid, it gives cobyrinamide/cobyramide (compound **21**), where partial removal of the ribose moiety from the phosphate gives (CN)$_2$Cbi–P **22**. Cobinic (R = OH) is formed by combining cobyrinic acid with D-1-

amino-2-propanol at position f, where hexaamide (R = NH_2) gives cobinamide. Cobamic acid (R = OH) is formed when cobinic acid is substituted at position 2 of aminopropanol by a-D-ribofuranose 3-phosphate, where its hexaamide (R = NH_2) is called cobamide. Complete hydrolysis of vitamin B_{12} (compound **1**) gives cobyrinic acid, $(CN)_2Cby$ **24**, (Fig. 3.4).

References

1. R. Banerjee, *Chemistry and Biochemistry of B_{12}*, John Wiley & Sons, New York, 1999.

2. P. A. Butler, S. Murtaza, B. Kräutler, Partial synthesis of $Co_\alpha Co_\beta$-dicyano-176-norcobinamide, *Monatsh. Chem.*, **137** (2006) 1579–1589.

3. Z. Schneider, *Comprehensive B_{12}: Chemistry, Biochemistry, Nutrition, Ecology, Medicine*, Walter deGruyter Inc., New York, 1987.

Chapter 4

B_{12} Organometallic Reactivity

4.1 Introduction

Organometallic compounds are defined as compounds containing a metal–carbon bond, R–M. Composites of Grignard reagents, that is Li and Mg, are amongst the most significant organic reagents. Several supplementary metals have been used, such as Cu, Na, Zn and Co, among others. Vitamin B_{12} was discovered and isolated 60 years ago, and as a crystallisable, red complex [1, 2], this was found as a cobalt complex of the remarkable corrin ligand, an exceptional member of the tetrapyrroles [3, 4]. In 1962 Lenhert and Hodgkin [5] reported the partial synthesis of vitamin B_{12} coenzymes and revealed the importance of a metal–carbon bond in enzymatic processes. Coenzyme B_{12} (Fig. 4.1) is, thus, recognised as an organometallic derivative of vitamin B_{12} [5]. In people, methionine synthase and methylmalonyl–CoA mutase use coenzyme B_{12} and methylcobalamin, correspondingly, B_{12} cofactors [6–8].

Corrinoids cross the outer membrane through the TonB-dependent transmembrane protein BtuB (Fig. 4.2).

In the periplasmatic space, substrates are trapped by BtuF and transferred to the cytoplasm via a translocation pathway formed by the inner membrane transporter $BtuC_2D_2F$ [9].

Molecular Modelling of Vitamin B_{12} and Its Analogues
Penny Poomani Govender, Francis Opoku, Olaide Olalekan Wahab,
and Ephraim Muriithi Kiarii
Copyright © 2022 Jenny Stanford Publishing Pte. Ltd.
ISBN 978-981-4877-58-9 (Hardcover), 978-1-003-21339-0 (eBook)
www.jennystanford.com

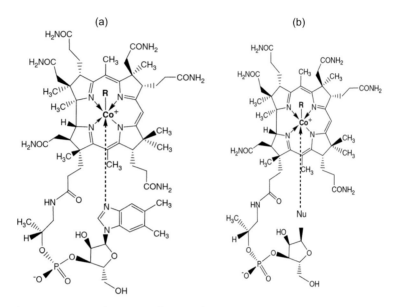

Figure 4.1 General structural formula. (a) Cobalamins (Cbls = DMB-cobamides, Ado = adenosyl). Vitamin B_{12} (1, CNCbl, R = CN), coenzyme B_{12} (2, R = 5′-deoxy-5′-ado), methylcobalamin (3, MeCbl, R = CH_3), aquacobalamin (4$^+$, R = H_2O^+), hydroxocobalamin (5, HOCbl, R = HO), cob(II)alamin (6, B_{12r}, R = e_), chlorocobalamin (18, R = Cl), nitroxylcobalamin (19, R = NO), 2,3-dihydroxypropyl-Cbl (21, R = 2,3-dihydroxy-propyl), α-adenosyl-Cbl (22, R = 50-deoxy-50-α-Ado), adeninylpropyl-Cbl (23, R = 3-adeninyl-propyl), homocoenzyme B_{12} (24, R = 50-deoxy-50-Ado-methyl), trifluoromethyl-Cbl (25, R = CF_3), difluoromethyl-Cbl (26, R = CHF_2), vinylcobalamin (28, R = CH=CH_2), cis-chlorovinyl-Cbl (29, R = CH=CHCl), bishomocoenzyme B_{12} (33, R = 2-[50-deoxy-50-Ado]-ethyl), 20-deoxycoenzyme B_{12} (48, R = 2′,5′-dideoxy-50-Ado) and 20,30-dideoxycoenzyme B_{12} (49, R = 20,30,50-trideoxy-50-Ado). (b) Structural formulae of other naturally occurring 'complete' corrinoids (cobamides with other nucleotide functions 'Nu' [6,11]: Cobcyano-imidazolylcobamide (14, R = CN, Nu = imidazole), cob-methyl-imidazolylcobamide (27, R = CH_3, Nu = imidazole), pseudovitamin B12 (cob-cyano-700-adeninylcobamide, 16, R = CN, Nu = adenine) and factor A (cob-cyano-700-[20-methyl]-adeninyl-cobamide, 17, R = CN, Nu = 2-methyladenine).

Organometallic compounds offer nucleophilic carbon atoms which react with electrophilic carbon, making a new carbon–carbon bond. This finds application in the creation of complex molecules from simple initial materials. To explain the general reactivity of organometallics it is expedient to view them as ionic, so R–M = R⁻M⁺. Like small organometallic compounds (Fig. 4.3), large ones react in a similar manner with electron-rich or anionic carbon atoms, that is as carbanions, which means they will function as either bases or nucleophiles.

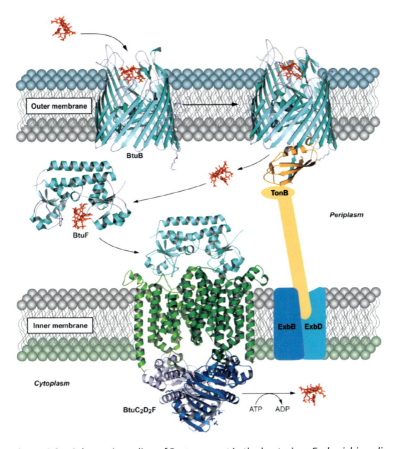

Figure 4.2 Schematic outline of B$_{12}$ transport in the bacterium *Escherichia coli*.

It is reasonable to think of these organometallic compounds as R⁻M⁺.

$$R\frown\!\!-H \rightleftarrows R\!:^- \ H^+$$

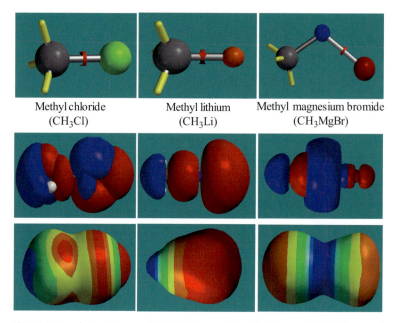

Figure 4.3 Electrostatic potentials for methyl chloride, methyl lithium and methyl magnesium bromide. The redder an area, the higher the electron density, and the bluer an area, the lower the electron density. In the alkyl halide, the methyl group has a lower electron density (blue) and is an electrophile.

4.2 Cobaloxime Model Systems

4.2.1 Formation of CoX Bonds

Alkylcobaloximes are used as simple models for the reactions of cobalamin-dependent enzymes. Reductive arylation has been used to secure the substituted arylcobaloximes (R = p-CF$_3$-C$_6$H$_4$, m- and p-MeO$_2$C*C$_6$H$_4$ or p-Ac*C$_6$H$_4$,). The alkylcobalamins are commonly prepared by alkylation of vitamin B$_{12s}$ with a primary alkyl halide or with an activated alkene, by reaction of B$_{12b}$ (hydroxocobalamin) with an enol ether, by reaction of non-activated alkenes (or alkyl bromides) with hydridocobalamin or by reaction of alkyl radicals with vitamin B$_{12r}$ under 'oxidising reducing' conditions. The preparations of methylcobalamin, hydroxocobalamin, (2,2-diethoxyethyl)cobalamin and aquamethylcobyrinic acid heptamethyl ester perchlorate have been described in detail [10]. The synthesis of alkylcobalamins from alkanes and vitamin B_{12r} under 'oxidising reducing' conditions has been extended to include the preparation of n-alkyl-, neopentyl-, isobutyl- and cycloalkylcobalamins from n-alkanes, neopentane, isobutane and cycloalkanes, respectively.

B_{12r} was found to react with alkyl halides. The kinetics of the reactions with alkyl chlorides and bromides conform to a second-order rate law which is interpreted in terms of a stepwise atom transfer mechanism (Eq. 4.1). On the other hand, the data for alkyl iodides are fitted by a third-order rate law which is consistent with an associative mechanism (Eq. 4.2) [11]. e-Adenosylcobalamin (synthesis and characterisation of 8-methoxy-5' deoxyadenosylcobalamin, a coenzyme B_{12} analogue which, following Co–C bond homolysis, avoids cyclisation of the 8-methoxy-5'-deoxyadenosyl radical) has been further studied [12].

$$B_{12r} + RX \xrightarrow[\substack{\text{rate} \\ \text{determining}}]{} XB_{12} + R^{\cdot} \; ; \; B_{12r} + R^{\cdot} \xrightarrow{\text{fast}} RB_{12}$$

$$XB_{12} + H_2O \longrightarrow B_{12a} + X^- \tag{4.1}$$

$$B_{12r} + RI \underset{\substack{\text{rapid} \\ \text{equillibrium}}}{\rightleftharpoons} [B_{12r}^{\cdot} RI] \; ; \; [B_{12r}^{\cdot} RI] + B_{12r} \xrightarrow{\text{rate determining}} RB_{12} + RB_{12a} + I^-$$

$$\tag{4.2}$$

4.2.2 Cleavage of Co–C Bonds

The Co–C bond dissociation energy of alkylcobalamins including co-enzyme B_{12} has been estimated to be in the range of $20–30$ kcal mol^{-1} Sterically hindered secondary alkylcobalamins with a β-hydrogen decompose spontaneously [13], under both anaerobic and aerobic conditions, by syn-elimination. However, in neutral aqueous solution under strictly anaerobic conditions, organylcobalamins which lack hydrogen in the P-position (namely neopentyl [13, 14] and benzyl [13] derivatives) decompose slowly by homolysis of the Co–C bond, since recombination of vitamin B_{12r} and organic radicals occurs with high efficiency. On the other hand, under aerobic conditions and in the presence of thiols, alcohols and imidazole, rapid oxidation or reaction of the radical species occurs [14]. It is suggested that the

B_{12} Organometallic Reactivity

homolytic cleavage is also triggered by upward distortions of the corrin ligand in response to re-coordination of the axial base [13]. The importance of distortions to the Co–C^α–X^β bond angle and Co–C^β bond length are explained by Baldwin et al. [14].

The thermodynamic method for the determination of metal-alkyl group bond dissociation energies, has been applied to two series of α-phenylethylcobaloximes, one containing 4-substituted pyridines as the axial base [15] and the other containing substituted phosphines of varying cone angles [16]. In the former case the Co–C bond dissociation energies increase systematically with the increase of the basicity of the ligand [15], and in the latter case the bond dissociation energies decrease dramatically as the cone angle of the phosphine increases [16]. The thermodynamic method has been augmented by a kinetic method [17] which involves the determination of the enthalpy of activation of the thermally induced homolytic process (Scheme 4.1). Based on the valid assumption that the enthalpy of activation of the reverse process is small, the bond dissociation energy can be estimated [18].

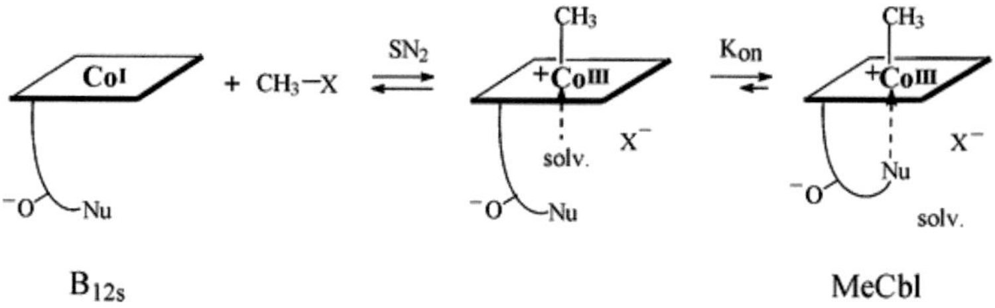

Scheme 4.1 Methylation of cob(I)alamin $B_{12}s$ (39) by an SN2 mode is directed to the 'upper' b-face (by both kinetic and thermodynamic reasons) and yields MeCbl (3).

These methods, which promise to have a wide application, have been reviewed [19, 20]. The factors influencing Co–C bond dissociation energies are of considerable importance for coenzyme B_{12}–dependent enzymatic processes [21–23].

4.2.3 Electrochemistry

Electrochemistry is an excellent method for the selective and controlled production of reduced B_{12} forms under potentiostat control. As alkyl halides or alkyl tosylates react quickly and efficiently with Co(I)-corrins [24], which are cleanly generated at controlled electrode potentials near that of Co(II)/Co(I) couples, electrochemistry provides a suitable method for the synthesis of organometallic B_{12} derivatives [25].

The polarographic electroreduction of aquocobalamin (B_{12a}) in acidic medium is complicated by adsorption of protonated B_{12r} at the dropping mercury electrode [10, 26]. A spectroelectrochemical study of cyanocobalamin reveals two closely separated one-electron reduction steps (Co (III) → Co (II) → Co (I)). However, at low electron flux, the reduction proceeds via one two-electron step because the reduction of 'base-off' B_{12r} is rapid compared to the reduction of B_{12}. Moreover, in the presence of added cyanide, the two reduction processes become successive again because cyanocob(II)alamin reduces more slowly than 'base-off' B_{12r} [27]. This behaviour may well be typical of other strong field ligands. The redox equilibrium properties of the Co III /Co II and Co II/Co I couples of diaquocobinamide are similar to those of the corresponding 'base-off' aquocobalamins [27]. Indeed, the one-electron reduction of organometallic Co(III)-corrins typically occurs at more negative potentials than the Co(II)/Co(I) redox couple B_{12r}/B_{12s} [25]. Using electrolysis at a controlled potential of –1.1 V versus the saturated calomel electrode (SCE), coenzyme B_{12} (2) was prepared in 95% yield from vitamin B_{12} (1) or from aquacobalamin (4^+) by alkylating cob(I)alamin (39^-) with 5'-chloro-5'-deoxyadenosine [28]. Other organometallic B_{12} derivatives produced in an analogous method were, for example pseudocoenzyme B_{12} (37) (78% yield from pseudovitamin B_{12}) [110], neocoenzyme B_{12} (39) (89% yield from neovitamin B_{12}) [29] and homocoenzyme B_{12} (24) (99% yield from 41) [30]. Cob-methyl-imidazolylcobamide (31) (90% yield from cob-cyano-imidazolylcobamide) [94] and methyl-13-epicob(III)alamin (46) (88% yield from neovitamin B_{12}) [29] were synthesised by alkylation with methyl iodide. Also, dimeric B_{12} derivatives, such as the cob-alkyl-bridged and sterically crowded tetramethylene-cob-1,4-biscobalamin (30) [31] and a strained organometallic B_{12}-rotaxane [32], were synthesised by similar methods (Fig. 4.4).

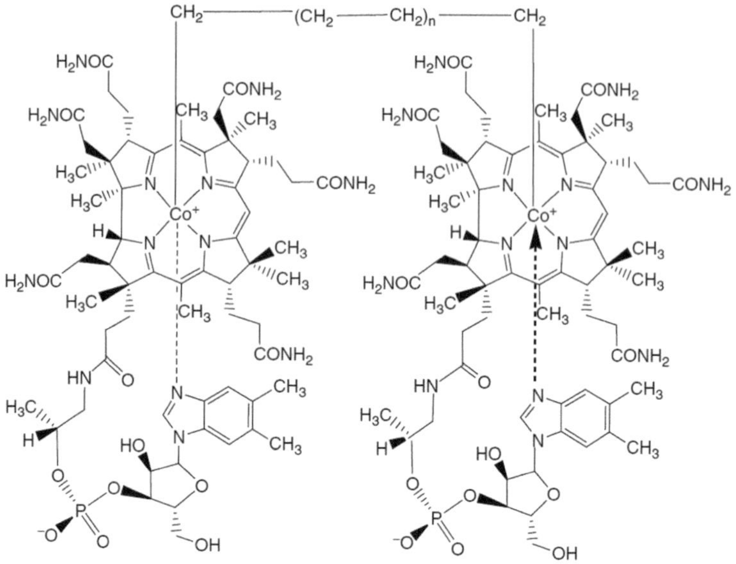

28 | B_{12} Organometallic Reactivity

Figure 4.4 Electrochemistry as a means for the preparation of alkyl-bridged biscorrinoids. Structural formulae of tetramethylene-bridged biscobalamin (30, $n = 1$) [24] and of a dodecamethylene-bridged biscobalamin ($n = 5$); symbolic representations of alkyl-bridged biscobalamins and of a cyclodextrin-based B_{12}-rotaxane [28].

Bimolecular homolytic displacement of benzylcobaloxime with a liphaticradicals yields benzylalkanes [33]. Oximes react photochemically with trichloromethylsulphonyl chloride to give high yields of alkanesulphonyl chloride [34]. The scope of the regiospecifically transfer reactions from substituted allyl cobaloximes to a variety of bromodiesters has been further explored [35].

4.2.4 Alkene Coupling

Vitamin B_{12} (1) benzyl radicals are formed from styrene derivatives, which furnish the respective dimers. Styrene derivatives, with (CN)Cbl (1a)/Ti(III) citrate, have been prepared by van der Donk using this methodology [36]. Van der Donk et al. revealed that the vitamin B_{12} precatalyst is first reduced by Ti (III) citrate to the catalytically active cob(I)alamin, which displays a characteristic purple colour with a UV maximum near 380 nm. The reduced metal catalyst activates the substrate to generate the stabilised radical *I*. Most likely the activation involves an inner sphere process which may involve an organocobalamin, followed by homolytic cleavage of the Co–C bond to produce *I* [36]. Radical *I* subsequently reacts intramolecularly with the alkene to generate radical *II*. The fate of this radical is dependent on the reaction conditions. It can either be reduced to yield product *III*, or cob(II)alamin can abstract a β-hydrogen atom to give the unsaturated product *IV*. This would also produce hydridocobalamin, which would be rapidly deprotonated (pK$_a$ ca. 1) [37], regenerating the active cob(I)alamin catalyst. Several studies have provided strong support for such a homolytic mechanism for the generation of alkenes as opposed to a β-hydride elimination mechanism from an alkylcobalamin species. An intramolecular reaction with dienes leads to the making of tetrahydrofuran derivatives, depending on the pH of the reaction mixture [38]. The light-induced methodology also works well for dimerising substituted styrenes (Scheme 4.2) [39].

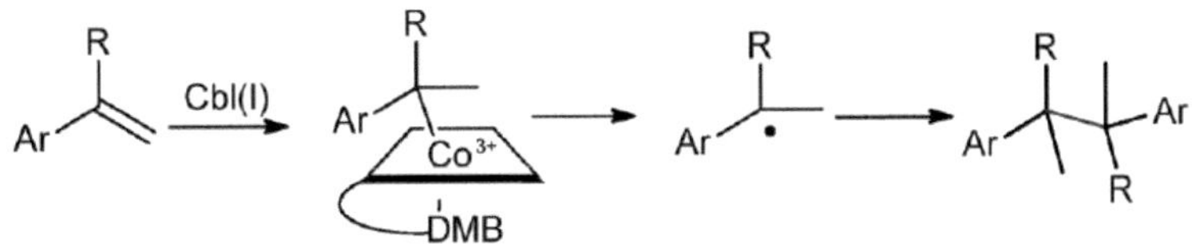

Scheme 4.2 General pathway for B$_{12}$-catalysed homocoupling of styrene derivatives.

4.2.5 Ring Expansion Reactions

Ring expansion reactions are significant in the making of cyclic compounds, mainly those which are challenging to access by other methods. Typically, ring expansions operate by migrating to an exocyclic leaving group (e.g., Tiffeneau–Demjanov rearrangement) or by forming and opening a bicyclic intermediate (e.g., Buchner reaction). The latter pathway was suggested by Dowd for a one-carbon ring expansion of cyclic α-(bromomethyl)-β-keto esters. A radical mechanism for this process was also proposed [40]. The application of Bu$_3$SnH as a radical promoter for ring expansion reactions is significantly limited in organic synthesis because numerous side reactions may occur. In contrast, cobalamin derivatives provide a gentler, greener alternative. Cby(II)(OMe)$_7$ could electrochemically form a Co(III)–alkyl complex which after homolysis generated a radical, which rearranged to afford a ring-expanded product (Scheme 4.3) [40]. The ring size strongly influences the reactivity of different substrates. Eight-membered rings have the lowest reactivity.

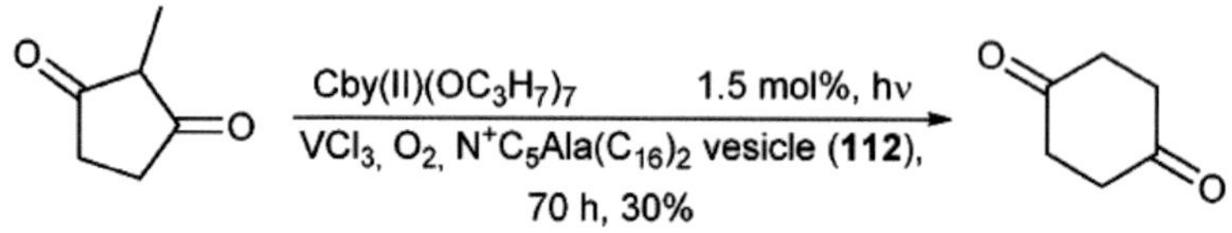

Scheme 4.3 Ring expansion of nonhalogenated cyclopentanedione, catalysed by Cby(II)(OC$_3$H$_7$)$_7$.

The ring expansion of cyclic α-(bromomethyl)-β-keto esters by one carbon unit has been examined rather extensively by generating radical species with Bu$_3$SnH [41–43]. Torii et al. have investigated ring expansion reactions of 2-alkyl-2-(bromomethyl) cycloalkanones, which have 5- and 6-membered rings, mediated by cobaloxime in methanol at 55°C–60°C by constant-current electrolysis under irradiation with visible light [44]. Other ring expansion reactions can apply to vitamin B$_{12}$ derivatives. [Cob(II)7C$_1$ester]ClO$_4$ was utilised to catalyse ring expansion reactions under conditions of controlled-potential electrolysis.

4.3 Computational Studies on Organometallic Chemistry

Computational studies have played a vital role in advancing our understanding of the electronic structures and catalytic cycles of bioorganometallic enzyme active sites and cofactors. While the success in obtaining high-resolution X-ray structures has permitted detailed insight into the coordination environments of the metal centres in these species, in many cases delivering surprising information regarding the composition of polynuclear metal clusters and revealing the identities of unusual active-site ligands, these structures often raised more questions concerning the corresponding catalytic mechanisms than they answered.

Therefore, computational studies – when properly evaluated on the basis of the results obtained in X-ray crystallographic, kinetic and/or spectroscopic investigations – will undoubtedly continue to play a key role in future research into the reaction cycles of the bioorganometallic systems. Computational approaches have been utilised with increasing frequency because they have proven to be an extremely useful complement to experimental investigations. For example, computations have been successfully used to investigate the formation and cleavage of the Co–C bond in a cobalamin comprehensive review in 2001 [45]. Several research groups have engaged in theoretical studies which were aimed at elucidating the molecular mechanism of Co–C bond activation by adenosylcobalamin-dependent enzymes [46–62]. The energy of Co–C bond heterolysis was found to decrease as a function of the trans Co–N bond length [53]. Moreover, evidence for the existence of a long axial ligand–Co bond opposite to the Co–CH$_3$ bond has been obtained for at least one member of the family of methyltransferases. To evaluate putative catalytic intermediates in methyl-coenzyme M (methyl-CoM) reductase, Siegbahn and coworkers [63, 64] computed the Ni–S bond strength of 39 kcal/mol for the putative CoM-S-Ni(II)F$_{430}$ species which is formed in this process, which is much closer to the 70 kcal/mol needed to cleave the S–C bond in methyl-CoM. The electron distributions and exchange interactions was observed to be the active site metal ions in carbon monoxide dehydrogenase/acetyl-coenzyme A synthase [65, 66] and the magnetic properties of the [FeFe] hydrogenase active-site cluster [67–69] was calculated. Computational approaches to chemistry are the prediction of energies and molecular geometries. There is a diverse selection of computational methods available to compute the electronic structure of a system at a fixed geometry. A typical geometry optimisation strategy can be illustrated by considering the Co–C bond of methylcobalamin [70]. First, a reasonable initial guess is made for the Co–C bond length and the total energy of methylcobalamin is computed for this particular nuclear configuration. To interpret the changes in terms of geometric and electronic structural perturbations of Co^{2+} cobalamin, researchers have used spectroscopically validated DFT computations as the basis for developing a spectro/structural correlation – specifically, a series of DFT and time-dependent DFT calculations to predict how distortions of the axial ligand–Co^{2+} bonding interaction affect the electronic absorption, magnetic circular dichroism and electron paramagnetic resonance spectra of Co^{2+} cobalamin [71, 72]. This correlation has enabled us to interpret the observed spectral changes accompanying the binding of Co^{2+} cobalamin to adenosyltransferase complexed with adenosine-5′-triphosphate in terms of the formation of an essentially four-coordinate Co^{2+} cobalamin species which lacks any significant axial bonding interactions [72, 73].

References

1. E. L. Rickes, N. G. Brink, F. R. Koniuszy, T. R. Wood, K. Folkers, Crystalline vitamin B_{12}, *Science*, **107** (1948) 396–397.

2. E. L. Smith, L. Parker, Purification of anti-pernicious anaemia factor, *Biochem. J.*, **43** (1947) viii.

3. D. C. Hodgkin, J. Pickworth, J. H. Robertson, K. N. Trueblood, R. J. Prosen, J. G. White, Structure of vitamin B_{12}: the crystal structure of the hexacarboxylic acid derived from B_{12} and the molecular structure of the vitamin, *Nature*, **176** (1955) 325–328.

4. D. C. Hodgkin, J. Kamper, M. Mackay, J. Pickworth, K. N. Trueblood, J. G. White, Structure of vitamin B_{12}, *Nature*, **178** (1956) 64–66.

5. P. G. Lenhert, D. C. Hodgkin, Structure of the 5, 6-dimethylbenzimidazolylcobamide coenzyme, *Nature*, **192** (1961) 937–938.

6. J. M. Pratt, *Inorganic Chemistry of Vitamin B_{12}*, Academic Press, London, UK, 1972.

7. T. K. Mazumder, N. Nishio, M. Hayashi, S. Nagai, Production of corrinoids including vitamin B-12 by *Methanosarcina barkeri* growing on methanol, *Biotechnol. Lett.*, **8** (1986) 843–848.

8. K. L. Brown, Chemistry and enzymology of vitamin B_{12}, *Chem. Rev.*, **105** (2005) 2075–2150.

9. K. Gruber, B. Puffer, B. Kräutler, Vitamin B_{12}-derivatives-enzyme cofactors and ligands of proteins and nucleic acids, *Chem. Soc. Rev.*, 40 (2011) 4346–4363.

10. B. Ridge, Organometallic compounds in biological chemistry, *Organomet. Chem.*, **11** (1983) 387.

11. H.-U. Blaser, J. Halpern, Reactions of vitamin B_{12r} with organic halides, *J. Am. Chem. Soc.*, **102** (1980) 1684–1689.

12. K. M. Doll, P. E. Fleming, R. G. Finke, The synthesis and characterization of 8-methoxy-5′-deoxyadenosylcobalamin: a coenzyme B_{12} analog which, following Co-C bond homolysis, avoids cyclization of the 8-methoxy-5′-deoxyadenosyl radical, *J. Inorg. Biochem.*, **91** (2002) 388–397.

13. G. N. Schrauzer, J. H. Grate, Sterically induced, spontaneous cobalt-carbon bond homolysis and .beta.-elimination reactions of primary and secondary organocobalamins, *J. Am. Chem. Soc.*, **103** (1981) 541–546.

14. D. A. Baldwin, E. A. Betterton, S. M. Chemaly, J. M. Pratt, The chemistry of vitamin B_{12}. Part 25. Mechanism of the β-elimination of olefins from alkylcorrinoids; evidence for an initial homolytic fission of the Co-C bond, *Dalton Trans.*, (1985) 1613–1618.

15. F. T. Ng, G. L. Rempel, C. Mancuso, J. Halpern, Decomposition of .alpha.-phenethylbis (dimethylglyoximato) cobalt (III) complexes. Influence of electronic and steric factors on the kinetics and thermodynamics of cobalt-carbon bond dissociation, *Organometallics*, **9** (1990) 2762–2772.

16. F. T. Ng, G. L. Rempel, J. Halpern, Steric influences on cobalt-alkyl bond dissociation energies, *Inorg. Chim. Acta*, **77** (1983) L165–L166.

17. T. T. Tsou, M. Loots, J. Halpern, Kinetic determination of transition metal-alkyl bond dissociation energies: application to organocobalt compounds related to B_{12} coenzymes, *J. Am. Chem. Soc.*, **104** (1982) 623–624.

18. R. G. Finke, B. L. Smith, B. J. Mayer, A. A. Molinero, Cobalt-cobalt bond homolysis and bond dissociation energy studies for the coenzyme B_{12} analog RCo [C_2(DO)(DOH)pn] I (R = $PhCH_2$-, $(CH_3)_3CCH_2$-), *Inorg. Chem.*, **22** (1983) 3677–3679.

19. J. Halpern, Determination and significance of transition metal-alkyl bond dissociation energies, *Acc. Chem. Res.*, **15** (1982) 238–244.

20. J. Halpern, Mechanistic aspects of coenzyme B_{12}-dependent rearrangements. Organometallics as free radical precursors, *Pure Appl. Chem.*, **55** (1983) 1059–1068.

21. D. R. Rao, M. C. Symons, Mechanisms for the photolysis and radiolysis of alkylcobaloximes and related compounds. An electron spin resonance study, *J. Chem. Soc., Faraday Trans. 1*, **80** (1984) 423–434.

22. M. Hoshino, S. Konishi, Y. Terai, M. Imamura, Optical and ESR studies of one-electron reduction of alkylcobaloximes in rigid matrixes, *Inorg. Chem.*, **21** (1982) 89–93.

23. H. Y. Al-Saigh, T. J. Kemp, Sensitization and quenching processes of alkylcobalt (III) compounds, *J. Chem. Soc., Perkin Trans. 2*, **2** (1983) 615–619.

24. R. Banerjee, *Chemistry and Biochemistry of B_{12}*, John Wiley & Sons, 1999.

25. D. Lexa, J. M. Saveant, The electrochemistry of vitamin B_{12}, *Acc. Chem. Res.*, **16** (1983) 235–243.

26. C. Schmidt, C. Kolpin, H. Swofford, Electrochemical behavior of the vitamin B_{12a}/vitamin B_{12r} couple on mercury and platinum electrodes, *Anal. Chem.*, **53** (1981) 41–47.

27. D. Lexa, J. Sayeant, J. Zickler, Electrochemistry of vitamin B_{12}. 5. Cyanocobalamins, *J. Am. Chem. Soc.*, **102** (1980) 2654–2663.

28. B. Kräutler, Organometallic chemistry of B_{12} coenzymes, *Met. Ions Life Sci.*, **6** (2009) 1–51.

29. G. Kontaxis, D. Riether, R. Hannak, M. Tollinger, B. Kräutler, Electrochemical synthesis and structure analysis of neocoenzyme B_{12}- an epimer of coenzyme B_{12} with a remarkably flexible organometallic group, *Helv. Chim. Acta*, **82** (1999) 848–869.

30. S. Gschösser, R. B. Hannak, R. Konrat, K. Gruber, C. Mikl, C. Kratky, B. Kräutler, Homocoenzyme B_{12} and bishomocoenzyme B_{12}: covalent structural mimics for homolyzed, enzyme-bound coenzyme B_{12}, *Chem. Eur. J.*, **11** (2005) 81–93.

31. B. Kräutler, T. Dérer, P. Liu, W. Mühlecker, M. Puchberger, K. Gruber, C. Kratky, Oligomethylene-bridged vitamin B_{12} dimers, *Angew. Chem. Int. Ed.*, **34** (1995) 84–86.

32. R. B. Hannak, G. Färber, R. Konrat, B. Kräutler, An organometallic B_{12}- rotaxane and a B_{12}-dimer, relaxed and loaded forms of a molecular spring, *J. Am. Chem. Soc.*, **119** (1997) 2313–2314.

33. R. McHatton, J. H. Espenson, A. Bakac, Reactions of aliphatic radicals and benzyl (aqua) cobaloxime: kinetics of coupling reactions as studied by novel kinetic competition methods, *J. Am. Chem. Soc.*, **104** (1982) 3531–3533.

34. P. Bougeard, M. D. Johnson, G. M. Lampman, Synthesis of alkanesulphonyl chlorides from alkylcobaloximes and trichloromethanesulphonyl chloride, *J. Chem. Soc., Perkin Trans. 1*, (1982) 849–854.

35. M. Veber, A. Gaudemer, M. Johnson, Reactions of organocobalt complexes with bromoesters: regiospecific synthesis of allyl- and cyclopropylmethyl-substituted malonic and acetoacetic esters, *J. Organomet. Chem.*, **209** (1981) 393–399.

36. J. Shey, C. M. McGinley, K. M. McCauley, A. S. Dearth, B. T. Young, W. A. Van der Donk, Mechanistic investigation of a novel vitamin B_{12}-catalyzed carbon-Carbon bond forming reaction, the reductive dimerization of arylalkenes, *J. Org. Chem.*, **67** (2002) 837–846.

37. M. D. Waddington, R. G. Finke, Neopentylcobalamin (neopentyl B_{12}) cobalt-carbon bond thermolysis products, kinetics, activation parameters, and bond dissociation energy: a chemical model exhibiting 106 of the 1012 enzymic activation of coenzyme B_{12}'s cobalt-carbon bond, *J. Am. Chem. Soc.*, **115** (1993) 4629–4640.

38. C. M. McGinley, H. A. Relyea, W. A. Van Der Donk, Vitamin B_{12} catalyzed radical cyclizations of arylalkenes, *Synlett*, **2006** (2006) 211–214.

39. H. Shimakoshi, Y. Hisaeda, B_{12}-TiO_2 hybrid catalyst for light-driven hydrogen production and hydrogenation of C–C multiple bonds, *ChemPlusChem*, **79** (2014) 1250–1253.

40. Y. Hisaeda, T. Nishioka, Y. Inoue, K. Asada, T. Hayashi, Electrochemical reactions mediated by vitamin B_{12} derivatives in organic solvents, *Coord. Chem. Rev.*, **198** (2000) 21–37.

41. P. Dowd, S. C. Choi, A new tributyltin hydride-based rearrangement of bromomethyl .beta.-keto esters. A synthetically useful ring expansion to .gamma.-keto esters, *J. Am. Chem. Soc.*, **109** (1987) 3493–3494.

42. P. Dowd, S. C. Choi, Free radical ring expansion by three and four carbons, *J. Am. Chem. Soc.*, **109** (1987) 6548–6549.

43. P. Dowd, S.-C. Choi, Novel free radical ring-expansion reactions, *Tetrahedron*, **45** (1989) 77–90.

44. T. Inokuchi, M. Tsuji, H. Kawafuchi, S. Torii, Indirect electroreduction of 2-alkyl-2-(bromomethyl) cycloalkanones with cobaloxime to form 3-alkyl-2-alkenones via 1, 2-acyl migration, *J. Org. Chem.*, **56** (1991) 5945–5948.

45. P. M. Kozlowski, Quantum chemical modeling of Co–C bond activation in B_{12}-dependent enzymes, *Curr. Opin. Chem. Biol.*, **5** (2001) 736–743.

46. R. Banerjee, A. Dybala-Defratyka, P. Paneth, Quantum catalysis in B_{12}-dependent methylmalonyl-CoA mutase: experimental and computational insights, *Philos. Trans. R. Soc. London, Ser. B*, **361** (2006) 1333–1339.

47. K. L. Brown, The enzymatic activation of coenzyme B_{12}, *Dalton Trans.*, (2006) 1123–1133.

48. A. J. Brooks, M. Vlasie, R. Banerjee, T. C. Brunold, Co–C bond activation in methylmalonyl-CoA mutase by stabilization of the post-homolysis product Co^{2+} cobalamin, *J. Am. Chem. Soc.*, **127** (2005) 16522–16528.

49. A. J. Brooks, C. C. Fox, E. N. G. Marsh, M. Vlasie, R. Banerjee, T. C. Brunold, Electronic structure studies of the adenosylcobalamin cofactor in glutamate mutase, *Biochemistry*, **44** (2005) 15167–15181.

50. A. J. Brooks, M. Vlasie, R. Banerjee, T. C. Brunold, Spectroscopic and computational studies on the adenosylcobalamin-dependent methylmalonyl-CoA mutase: evaluation of enzymatic contributions to Co–C bond activation in the Co^{3+} ground state, *J. Am. Chem. Soc.*, **126** (2004) 8167–8180.

51. N. Dölker, A. Morreale, F. Maseras, Computational study on the difference between the Co–C bond dissociation energy in methylcobalamin and adenosylcobalamin, *J. Biol. Inorg. Chem.*, **10** (2005) 509–517.

52. N. Dölker, F. Maseras, P. E. Siegbahn, Stabilization of the adenosyl radical in coenzyme B_{12}–a theoretical study, *Chem. Phys. Lett.*, **386** (2004) 174–178.

53. N. Dölker, F. Maseras, A. Lledos, Density functional study on the effect of the trans axial ligand of B_{12} cofactors on the heterolytic cleavage of the Co–C bond, *J. Phys. Chem. B*, **107** (2003) 306–315.

54. K. P. Jensen, U. Ryde, How the Co–C bond is cleaved in coenzyme B_{12} enzymes: a theoretical study, *J. Am. Chem. Soc.*, **127** (2005) 9117–9128.

55. K. P. Jensen, U. Ryde, Theoretical prediction of the Co–C bond strength in cobalamins, *J. Phys. Chem. A*, **107** (2003) 7539–7545.

56. K. P. Jensen, S. P. Sauer, T. Liljefors, P.-O. Norrby, Theoretical investigation of steric and electronic effects in coenzyme B_{12} models, *Organometallics*, **20** (2001) 550–556.

57. M. Jaworska, P. Lodowski, T. Andruniów, P. M. Kozlowski, Photolysis of methylcobalamin: identification of the relevant excited states involved in Co–C bond scission, *J. Phys. Chem. B*, **111** (2007) 2419–2422.

58. J. Kuta, S. Patchkovskii, M. Z. Zgierski, P. M. Kozlowski, Performance of DFT in modeling electronic and structural properties of cobalamins, *J. Comput. Chem.*, **27** (2006) 1429–1437.

59. R. A. Kwiecien, I. V. Khavrutskii, D. G. Musaev, K. Morokuma, R. Banerjee, P. Paneth, Computational insights into the mechanism of radical generation in B_{12}-dependent methylmalonyl-CoA mutase, *J. Am. Chem. Soc.*, **128** (2006) 1287–1292.

60. A. Dybala-Defratyka, P. Paneth, R. Banerjee, D. G. Truhlar, Coupling of hydrogenic tunneling to active-site motion in the hydrogen radical transfer catalyzed by a coenzyme B_{12}-dependent mutase, *Proc. Natl. Acad. Sci.*, **104** (2007) 10774–10779.

61. P. M. Kozlowski, T. Kamachi, T. Toraya, K. Yoshizawa, Does Cob (II) alamin act as a conductor in coenzyme B_{12} dependent mutases?, *Angew. Chem. Int. Ed.*, **46** (2007) 980–983.

62. P. K. Sharma, Z. T. Chu, M. H. Olsson, A. Warshel, A new paradigm for electrostatic catalysis of radical reactions in vitamin B_{12} enzymes, *Proc. Natl. Acad. Sci.*, **104** (2007) 9661–9666.

63. V. Pelmenschikov, M. R. Blomberg, P. E. Siegbahn, R. H. Crabtree, A mechanism from quantum chemical studies for methane formation in methanogenesis, *J. Am. Chem. Soc.*, **124** (2002) 4039–4049.

64. V. Pelmenschikov, P. E. Siegbahn, Catalysis by methyl-coenzyme M reductase: a theoretical study for heterodisulfide product formation, *J. Biol. Inorg. Chem.*, **8** (2003) 653–662.

65. R. P. Schenker, T. C. Brunold, Computational studies on the A cluster of acetyl-coenzyme A synthase: geometric and electronic properties of the NiFeC species and mechanistic implications, *J. Am. Chem. Soc.*, **125** (2003) 13962–13963.

66. P. Amara, A. Volbeda, J. C. Fontecilla-Camps, M. J. Field, A quantum chemical study of the reaction mechanism of acetyl-coenzyme A synthase, *J. Am. Chem. Soc.*, **127** (2005) 2776–2784.

67. A. T. Fiedler, T. C. Brunold, Computational studies of the H-cluster of Fe-only hydrogenases: geometric, electronic, and magnetic properties and their dependence on the $[Fe_4S_4]$ cubane, *Inorg. Chem.*, **44** (2005) 9322–9334.

68. L. Noodleman, C. Peng, D. Case, J.-M. Mouesca, Orbital interactions, electron delocalization and spin coupling in iron-sulfur clusters, *Coord. Chem. Rev.*, **144** (1995) 199–244.

69. L. Noodleman, D. A. Case, Density-functional theory of spin polarization and spin coupling in iron-sulfur clusters, *Adv. Inorg. Chem.*, **38** (1992) 423–470.

70. L. Randaccio, M. Furlan, S. Geremia, M. Šlouf, I. Srnova, D. Toffoli, Similarities and differences between cobalamins and cobaloximes. Accurate structural determination of methylcobalamin and of LiCl- and KCl-containing cyanocobalamins by synchrotron radiation, *Inorg. Chem.*, **39** (2000) 3403–3413.

71. T. A. Stich, N. R. Buan, T. C. Brunold, Spectroscopic and computational studies of Co^{2+} corrinoids: spectral and electronic properties of the biologically relevant base-on and base-off forms of Co^{2+} cobalamin, *J. Am. Chem. Soc.*, **126** (2004) 9735–9749.

72. T. A. Stich, N. R. Buan, J. C. Escalante-Semerena, T. C. Brunold, Spectroscopic and computational studies of the ATP: corrinoid adenosyltransferase (CobA) from Salmonella enterica: insights into the mechanism of adenosylcobalamin biosynthesis, *J. Am. Chem. Soc.*, **127** (2005) 8710–8719.

73. T. A. Stich, M. Yamanishi, R. Banerjee, T. C. Brunold, Spectroscopic evidence for the formation of a four-coordinate Co^{2+} cobalamin species upon binding to the human ATP: cobalamin adenosyltransferase, *J. Am. Chem. Soc.*, **127** (2005) 7660–7661.

Chapter 5

Coenzyme B$_{12}$–Dependent Enzymes

5.1 Introduction

The B$_{12}$s, also referred to as cobalamin coenzymes, are complex macrocycles whose reactivity is associated with a unique cobalt–carbon bond. Carbon skeleton isomerases glutamate mutase, methylmalonyl-CoA mutase and 2-methyleneglutarate mutase; the isomerase lysine 5,6-aminomutase; the isomerases/eliminases propane-1,2-diol hydrolyase (dioldehydrase), glycerol hydrolyase (glycerol dehydrase) and ethanolamine ammonia-lyase; and the class II ribonucleoside triphosphate reductase form the main enzymes.

There are two biologically active forms, methylcobalamin (MeCbl) and adenosylcobalamin (AdoCbl) (Fig. 5.1), and their closely related cobamide forms. MeCbl participates as the intermediate carrier of activated methyl groups. During the catalytic cycle, the coenzyme shuttles between MeCbl and the highly nucleophilic cob(I)alamin form. Examples of MeCbl-dependent enzymes include methionine synthase and Me-H$_4$-MPT:coenzyme M (CoM) methyltransferase. AdoCbl functions as a source of carbon-based free radicals which are unmasked by homolysis of the coenzyme's cobalt–carbon bond. The free radicals are subsequently used to remove non-acid hydrogen atoms from substrates to facilitate a variety of reactions involving cleavage of carbon–carbon, carbon–oxygen and carbon–

Molecular Modelling of Vitamin B$_{12}$ and Its Analogues
Penny Poomani Govender, Francis Opoku, Olaide Olalekan Wahab,
and Ephraim Muriithi Kiarii
Copyright © 2022 Jenny Stanford Publishing Pte. Ltd.
ISBN 978-981-4877-58-9 (Hardcover), 978-1-003-21339-0 (eBook)
www.jennystanford.com

nitrogen bonds. Most reactions involve 1,2 migrations of hydroxy-, amino- and carbon-containing groups, but there is also one class of ribonucleotide reductases which uses AdoCbl. The structures of two cobalamin-dependent enzymes, methionine synthase and methylmalonyl-CoA mutase, have been solved. In both cases the cobalt is coordinated by a histidine ligand from the protein. The significance of this binding motif is presently unclear since in other cobalamin-dependent enzymes spectroscopic evidence suggests that the coenzyme's nucleotide 'tail' remains coordinated to cobalt when bound to the protein.

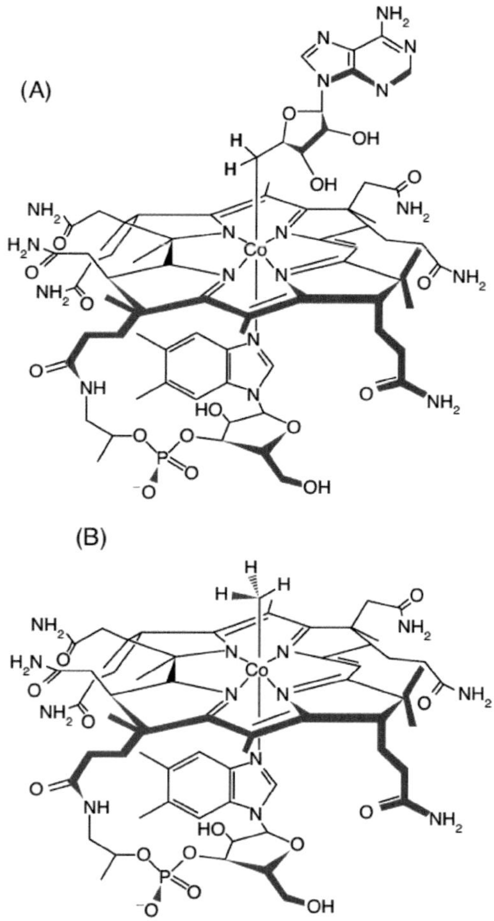

Figure 5.1 Structures of B_{12} coenzymes (A) adenosylcobalamin and (B) methylcobalamin [1].

Both MeCbl and AdoCbl play essential roles in the metabolism in higher eukaryotes [2]. In humans, lack of B_{12} in the diet, or an inability to absorb it, is the cause of pernicious anaemia. MeCbl is involved in the methylation of homocysteine to form methionine by methionine synthase as part of the methionine salvage pathway; homocysteine is toxic in high concentrations and may be responsible for many of the symptoms of pernicious anaemia. AdoCbl is the coenzyme for methylmalonyl-CoA mutase, an enzyme which converts methylmalonyl-CoA to succinyl-CoA, which is an essential step in the metabolism of odd-chain fatty acids [2]. The figure illustrates examples of Cbls with different β-coordinating ligands include CNCbl, H_2OCbl, MeCbl and AdoCbl (Fig. 5.2) [3], which originate from the occupation of the opposite, 'upper' (b)-site.

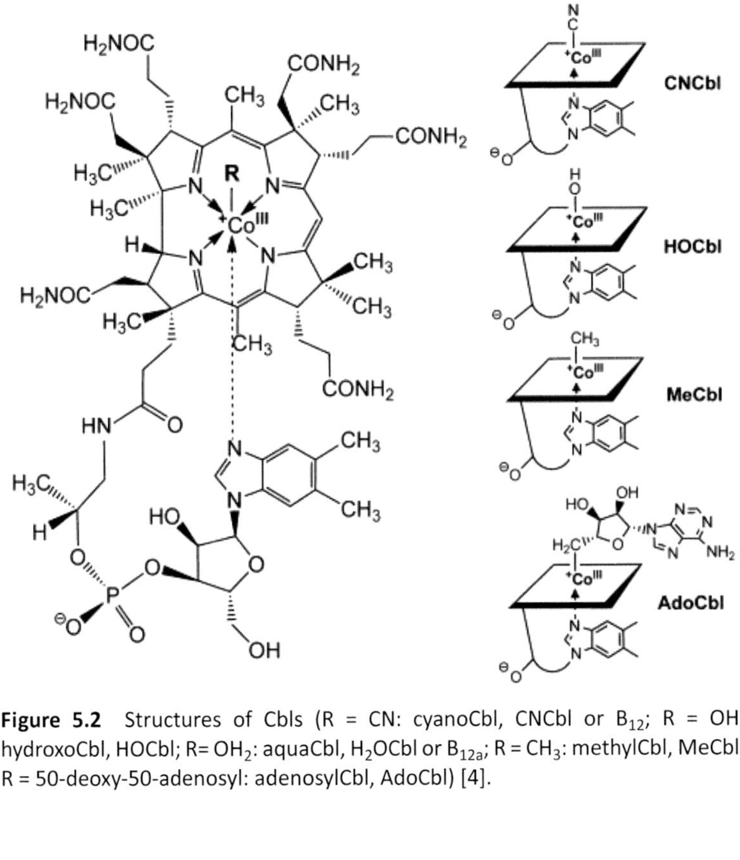

Figure 5.2 Structures of Cbls (R = CN: cyanoCbl, CNCbl or B_{12}; R = OH: hydroxoCbl, HOCbl; R= OH_2: aquaCbl, H_2OCbl or B_{12a}; R = CH_3: methylCbl, MeCbl; R = 50-deoxy-50-adenosyl: adenosylCbl, AdoCbl) [4].

5.2 Methylcobalamin

MeCbl is a form of vitamin B_{12} which features an octahedral cobalt(III) centre [5]. From the perspective of coordination chemistry, MeCbl is distinguished as an uncommon example of a compound which contains metal–alkyl bonds.

5.2.1 Methionine Synthase

Methionine synthase is a mammalian enzyme which metabolises 5-methyltetrahydrofolate to restore the dynamic cofactor tetrahydrofolate. In cobalamin-dependent forms of the enzyme, the reaction proceeds by two steps in a Ping-Pong reaction. The enzyme is initially primed into a reactive state by the transfer of a methyl group from 5-methyltetrahydrofolate to Co(I) in enzyme-bound cobalamin, forming methyl-cobalamin which now contains methyl-cobalamin(III) and activating the enzyme. Then, homocysteine which has coordinated to an enzyme-bound zinc to form a reactive thiolate reacts with the methyl-cobalamin. The activated methyl group is transferred from methyl-cobalamin to the homocysteine thiolate, which regenerates Co(I) in cob, and methionine is released from the enzyme. The cob-independent mechanism follows the same general pathway but with a direct reaction between the zinc thiolate and 5-methyltetrahydrofolate [6].

Methionine synthase is responsibly involved in converting homocysteine to methionine, encoded as 5-methyltetrahydrofolate-homocysteine methyltransferase in human beings [7]. It makes a portion of the S-adenosylmethionine [8]. Plants are cobalamin-independent [9]. Microorganisms have been found to have cobalamin-independent and cobalamin-dependent forms [9]. The enzyme catalyses the last step in the conversion of homocysteine to methionine. The reaction converts tetrahydrofolate to 5-methyltetrahydrofolate, changing a methyl group methionine to homocysteine form.

The mechanism of the enzyme depends on the constant regeneration of Co(I) in cob, but this is not always guaranteed. Instead, every 1–2000 catalytic turnovers, the Co(I) may be oxidised into Co(II), which would permanently shut down catalytic activity. A separate protein, methionine synthase reductase, catalyses the regeneration of Co(I) and the restoration of enzymatic activity.

Because the oxidation of cob-Co(I) inevitably shuts down cob-dependent methionine synthase activity, defects or deficiencies in methionine synthase reductase have been implicated in some of the disease associations for methionine synthase deficiency discussed later. The two enzymes form a scavenger network seen on the lower left [10]. Methionine synthase from *Escherichia coli* is the most further studied B_{12}-dependent enzyme [11].

5.2.2 Methylated-thiol-Coenzyme M Methyltransferase

Tallant et al.'s [12] study on the conversion of CoM methyltransferase ascribes that methanogenesis from dimethylsulphide requires the intermediate methylation of CoM. This reaction is catalysed by a methylthiol:CoM methyltransferase composed of two polypeptides, MtsA (a MeCbl:CoM methyltransferase) and MtsB (homologous to a class of corrinoid proteins involved in methanogenesis). Further studies have been done on the same subject [12–14] and show that methylated-thiol-CoM methyltransferase catalyses the chemical reaction of methanethiol and CoM to methyl CoM plus hydrogen sulphide as (1a) methanethiol and (Co(I) methylated-thiol-specific corrinoid protein) yields (methyl-Co(III) methylated-thiol-specific corrinoid protein) and hydrogen sulphide. In another reaction (1b) (methyl-Co(III) methylated-thiol-specific corrinoid protein) plus CoM gives methyl-CoM and (Co(I) methylated-thiol-specific corrinoid protein); this enzyme is involved in methanogenesis from methylated thiols, such as methanethiol, dimethyl sulphide and 3-S-methylmercaptopropionate.

One of the better-understood systems is the methanobacterium thermoautotrophicum methyltransferase, which catalyses the transfer of a methyl group from methyltetrahydromethanopterin to mercaptoethane sulphonate, a reaction chemically very similar to that catalysed by methionine synthase. Methyl-CoM is the substrate for methyl-CoM reductase which uses the nickel-containing macrocycle, coenzyme F450, to reduce the methyl group to methane and regenerate CoM [15]. Methyl-CoM reductase is the key enzyme of methane formation in methanogenic Archaea. It catalyses the reduction of methyl-CoM, CH_3-S-CoM, 2-(methylthio) ethanesulphonate, with coenzyme B (CoB) (CoB-S-H, 7-thioheptanoyl-threoninephosphate) to methane and the heterodisulphide of CoM (CoM-S-H, 2-thioethane sulphonate) and CoB under strictly anaerobic conditions [16, 17].

Spectroscopic investigations of methyl-CoM reductase have revealed several Ni electron paramagnetic resonance (EPR)-active and EPR-inactive states of the enzyme [18]. After harvesting of H_2–CO_2-grown cells, the enzyme is present in an inactive EPR silent state designated as MCR_{silent}. In this state, methyl-CoM reductase contains bound CoM [19] and coenzyme B (CoB) [20] and can only be partially reactivated by enzymatic reduction [21]. When cells are gassed with H_2 before harvesting, the enzyme is present in an active MCR_{red1} state whose characteristic Ni(I) F_{430} EPR spectrum, designated as red 1, can be correlated with the enzymatic activity in the enzyme [22].

5.3   Adenosylcobalamin

AdoCbl referred to as cobamamide and dibencozide is, along with MeCbl, an active form of vitamin B_{12}. Mainly available as a nutritional supplement, alongside MeCbl, hydroxocobalamin and cyanocobalamin, AdoCbl can catalyse both the migration of hydroxy or amino groups in vicinal diols or amino alcohols, followed by dehydration or deamination to yield aldehydes and, the aminomutases, which catalyse the 1,2 migration of an amino group within an amino acid and also require pyridoxal phosphate as an additional coenzyme.

5.4   Hydroxocobalamin

Hydroxocobalamin was used as an antidote in experimental cyanide poisoning in mice in 1952 [25] and has since been shown to be efficacious in a variety of animal models [26]. It has been used for the treatment of human cyanide poisoning in France since the 1970s [27, 28]. Hydroxocobalamin has also been used to treat smoke inhalation victims [29] and children poisoned by improperly prepared cassava [30]. In lower doses, it has been used to treat diseases thought to be caused by chronic, low-level cyanide exposure, tobacco amblyopia and Leber's hereditary optic atrophy [31].

Experimentally, hydroxocobalamin has been used as prophylaxis for cyanide poisoning during sodium nitroprusside therapy [27, 32]. Hydroxocobalamin detoxifies cyanide by giving up a hydroxyl group and binding a cyanyl group, forming nontoxic cyanocobalamin (vitamin B_{12}), which is excreted in the urine [28]. It does not have the problems inherent with sodium nitrite: profound hypotension from vasodilation and possible excessive induction of methemoglobinemia (undesirable in cases of combined carbon monoxide and cyanide poisoning from smoke inhalation or when the diagnosis is uncertain) [28, 33].

Hydroxocobalamin has further been used to treat cyanide poisoning [34], toxic amblyopia [35] and Leber's optic atrophy [36] and is commonly referred to as vitamin B_{12a}. The main source is found in food as well as often given as a supplement. Cobalamins together with folate are required in the formation of DNA at the chromosomal division and replication process. Hydroxocobalamin is altered to either 5-deoxyadenosyl cobalamin or MeCbl and serves as storage in the serum [37]

5.5 Cobamamide

Methylmalonyl-CoA mutase (MCM) enzyme uses cabamamide (dibencozide or AdoCbl) as a cofactor. Cabamamide is an active form of vitamin B_{12}. It has the formula $C_{72}H_{100}CoN_{18}O_{17}P$. Coenzyme B_{12} (5'-deoxyadenosylcobalamin), in which the configuration of the N-glycosidic bond in the Ado ligand is inverted (α-ribo) AdoCbl, has been synthesised and its crystal structure determined by X-ray diffraction, MoKα: λ = 0.71073 Å; monoclinic P212121; a = 16.132(12) Å, b = 21.684(15) Å, c = 27.30(3) Å; 9611 independent reflections; R1 = 0.0708. As suggested by molecular mechanics (MM) modelling before the structure was known, the Ado ligand lies over the southern quadrant of the molecule, as is the case for AdoCbl. The most striking feature of the structure is a disorder in the orientation of the adenine (Ade) moiety relative to the ribose of the Ado ligand. This was resolved with a two-state model in which in the major (0.57 occupancy) conformer the A16(O)-A11-A9(N)-A8 dihedral angle is 1.9° and the Ade is virtually perpendicular to the corrin ring; in the minor conformer, the Ade is tilted down, and this dihedral is −48.7°. The Co–C and axial Co–N bond lengths and the Co–C–C bond angle are quite similar to those in AdoCbl. The corrin ring is considerably flatter than that of AdoCbl, with a fold angle of 11.7°. The molecule was successfully modelled by MM, and rotation of the Ado ligand relative to the corrin gave rise to four locally minimum structures with the Ado in the southern, eastern, northern or western quadrant, with the southern conformation as the global minimum, as is the case with AdoCbl itself.

5.6   Cyanocobalamin

This is a synthetic form of vitamin B_{12} with the general formula of $C_{63}H_{88}CoN_{14}O_{14}P$, administered as an injection. Cob(III)alamin cyanide is a product of cob(I)alamin, cyanide, and $NADP^+$ (Eq. 5.1).

$$cob(I)alamin + cyanide + NADP^+ \rightleftharpoons cyanocob(III)alamin$$
$$+ NADPH + H^+ \quad (5.1)$$

The resultant three products are NADPH, H^+ and cyanocob(III) alamin. This enzyme originates from the classification of oxidoreductases, precisely the ones which oxidise metal ions and use $NADP^+$ or NAD^+ as an electron acceptor for the oxidisation reaction. The systematic name of this enzyme class is cob(I) alamin cyanide:$NADP^+$ oxidoreductase. Other names used describe the same include yanocobalamin reductase (NADPH, cyanide-eliminating), cyanocobalamin reductase, NADPH:cyanocob(III) alamin oxidoreductase (cyanide-eliminating) and ccyanocobalamin reductase (NADPH, CN-eliminating). The coenzyme is instable towards light and acid [38, 39]. The structure of the coenzyme was elucidated through the crystallographic studies of Hodgkin [39], who showed that the general macrocyclic structure and peripheral substituents were the same for both cyanocobalamin and the vitamin coenzyme and also demonstrated a unique feature of the coenzyme, the covalent bond between cobalt and the 5′ carbon of an adenine moiety. This was the first example of a naturally occurring organometallic compound. Indeed, to this day the vitamin coenzyme and related alkylcobalamins represent the only known organometallic compounds of nature [39].

While the crystallographic studies elucidated the major structural features of the cyanocobalamin coenzyme, they left open the possibility that the extent of the conjugated chromophore might be different in the coenzyme than that of B_{12} itself. This difference in the extent of oxidation of the chromophore was suggested by studies on the formation of the coenzyme from vitamin and would have been consistent with the considerable differences in the optical spectra of the coenzyme (orange-yellow) and B_{12} (red-purple) [39]. The degree of unsaturation of the corrin chromophore was related to, and further complicated by, the oxidation state of the cobalt, which is trivalent diamagnetic in vitamin B_{12} but which had been reported to be paramagnetic by some and diamagnetic by others in the coenzyme. At this time the coenzyme had been prepared by an initial reduction of cyano- or hydroxocobalamin, followed by alkylation with a suitable derivative of 5/-deoxyadenosine [39]. Thus the mode of formation did not define the oxidation state of the cobalt and allowed for the possible reduction of the chromophore during the formation of the coenzyme.

References

1. E. Marsh, Coenzyme B_{12} (cobalamin)-dependent enzymes, *Essays Biochem.*, **34** (1999) 139–154.
2. S. Savvi, D. F. Warner, B. D. Kana, J. D. McKinney, V. Mizrahi, S. S. Dawes, Functional characterization of a vitamin B_{12}-dependent methylmalonyl pathway in Mycobacterium tuberculosis: implications for propionate metabolism during growth on fatty acids, *J. Bacteriol.*, **190** (2008) 3886–3895.
3. G. Schrauzer, *Inorganic Chemistry of Vitamin B_{12}*, Academic Press, New York, USA, 1972.
4. B. Kräutler, Antivitamins B_{12}-a structure- and reactivity-based concept, *Chem. Eur. J.*, **21** (2015) 11280–11287.
5. W. T. Wangui, G. N. Kamau, M. S. Ngari, M. C. Njambi, Electrocatalytic reduction of 2, 2, 2-trichloro-1, 1-bis (4-chlorophenyl) ethanol (dicofol) in acetonitrile-aqueous solution using cyanocobalamin as a catalyst, *Science*, **3** (2015) 1–10.
6. R. G. Matthews, A. E. Smith, Z. S. Zhou, R. E. Taurog, V. Bandarian, J. C. Evans, M. Ludwig, Cobalamin-dependent and cobalamin-independent

methionine synthases: are there two solutions to the same chemical problem?, *Helv. Chim. Acta*, **86** (2003) 3939–3954.

7. Y. N. Li, S. Gulati, P. J. Baker, L. C. Brody, R. Banerjee, W. D. Kruger, Cloning, mapping and RNA analysis of the human methionine synthase gene, *Hum. Mol. Genet.*, **5** (1996) 1851–1858.

8. R. V. Banerjee, R. G. Matthews, Cobalamin-dependent methionine synthase, *FASEB J.*, **4** (1990) 1450–1459.

9. T. Zydowsky, L. Courtney, V. Frasca, K. Kobayashi, H. Shimizu, L. Yuen, R. Matthews, S. Benkovic, H. Floss, Stereochemical analysis of the methyl transfer catalyzed by cobalamin-dependent methionine synthase from *Escherichia coli B*, *J. Am. Chem. Soc.*, **108** (1986) 3152–3153.

10. K. R. Wolthers, N. S. Scrutton, Protein interactions in the human methionine synthase-methionine synthase reductase complex and implications for the mechanism of enzyme reactivation, *Biochemistry*, **46** (2007) 6696–6709.

11. M. L. Ludwig and, R. G. Matthews, Structure-based perspectives on B_{12}-dependent enzymes, *Annu. Rev. Biochem.*, **66** (1997) 269–313.

12. T. C. Tallant, L. Paul, J. A. Krzycki, The MtsA subunit of the methylthiol: coenzyme M methyltransferase of Methanosarcina barkeri catalyses both half-reactions of corrinoid-dependent dimethylsulfide: coenzyme M methyl transfer, *J. Biol. Chem.*, **276** (2001) 4485–4493.

13. L. Paul, J. A. Krzycki, Sequence and transcript analysis of a novel Methanosarcina barkeri methyltransferase II homolog and its associated corrinoid protein homologous to methionine synthase, *J. Bacteriol.*, **178** (1996) 6599–6607.

14. T. C. Tallant, J. A. Krzycki, Methylthiol: coenzyme M methyltransferase from Methanosarcina barkeri, an enzyme of methanogenesis from dimethylsulfide and methylmercaptopropionate, *J. Bacteriol.*, **179** (1997) 6902–6911.

15. U. Ermler, W. Grabarse, S. Shima, M. Goubeaud, R. K. Thauer, Crystal structure of methyl-coenzyme M reductase: the key enzyme of biological methane formation, *Science*, **278** (1997) 1457–1462.

16. R. Thauer, Biodiversity and unity in biochemistry, *Antonie van Leeuwenhoek*, **71** (1997) 21–32.

17. R. S. Wolfe, My kind of biology, *Annu. Rev. Microbiol.*, **45** (1991) 1–36.

18. S. Albracht, D. Ankel-Fuchs, R. Böcher, J. Ellermann, J. Moll, J. Van der Zwaan, R. Thauer, Five new EPR signals assigned to nickel in methyl-coenzyme M reductase from Methanobacterium thermoautotrophicum,

strain Marburg, *Biochim. Biophys. Acta, Protein Struct. Mol. Enzymol.*, **955** (1988) 86–102.

19. P. Hartzell, M. Donnelly, R. Wolfe, Incorporation of coenzyme M into component C of methylcoenzyme M methylreductase during in vitro methanogenesis, *J. Biol. Chem.*, **262** (1987) 5581–5586.

20. K. M. Noll, R. S. Wolfe, Component C of the methylcoenzyme M methylreductase system contains bound 7-mercaptoheptanoylthreonine phosphate (HS-HTP), *Biochem. Biophys. Res. Commun.*, **139** (1986) 889–895.

21. P. E. Rouvière, R. S. Wolfe, Component A3 of the methylcoenzyme M methylreductase system of Methanobacterium thermoautotrophicum delta H: resolution into two components, *J. Bacteriol.*, **171** (1989) 4556–4562.

22. S. Rospert, R. Böcher, S. Albracht, R. Thauer, Methyl-coenzyme M reductase preparations with high specific activity from H_2-preincubated cells of Methanobacterium thermoautotrophicum, *FEBS Lett.*, **291** (1991) 371–375.

23. D. Crowfoot-Hodgkin, Die Röntgenstrukturanalyse komplizierter Moleküle. Nobel-Vortrag am 12. Dezember 1964, *Angew. Chem.*, **77** (1965) 954–962.

24. K. Gruber, B. Puffer, B. Kräutler, Vitamin B_{12}-derivatives-enzyme cofactors and ligands of proteins and nucleic acids, *Chem. Soc. Rev.*, **40** (2011) 4346–4363.

25. C. W. Mushett, K. L. Kelley, G. E. Boxer, J. C. Rickards, Antidotal efficacy of vitamin B_{12a} (hydroxo-cobalamin) in experimental cyanide poisoning, *Proc. Soc. Exp. Biol. Med.*, **81** (1952) 234–237.

26. J. C. Linnell, The role of cobalamins in cyanide detoxification, in *Clinical and Experimental Toxicology of Cyanides*, eds. B. Ballantyne, T. C. Marrs, Wright Pub., Bristol (1987) pp. 427–439.

27. A. Brouard, B. Blaisot, C. Bismuth, Hydroxocobalamine in cyanide poisoning, *J. Toxicol. Clin. Exp.*, **7** (1987) 155–168.

28. J. C. Forsyth, P. D. Mueller, C. E. Becker, J. Osterloh, N. L. Benowitz, B. H. Rumack, A. H. Hall, Hydroxocobalamin as a cyanide antidote: safety, efficacy and pharmacokinetics in heavily smoking normal volunteers, *J. Toxicol.: Clin. Toxicol.*, **31** (1993) 277–294.

29. F. J. Baud, P. Barriot, V. Toffis, B. Riou, E. Vicaut, Y. Lecarpentier, R. Bourdon, A. Astier, C. Bismuth, Elevated blood cyanide concentrations in victims of smoke inhalation, *New Engl. J. Med.*, **325** (1991) 1761–1766.

30. O. Espinoza, M. Perez, M. Ramirez, Bitter cassava poisoning in eight children: a case report, *Vet. Hum. Toxicol.*, **34** (1992) 65.

31. C. Bismuth, F. Baud, P. Pontal, Hydroxocobalamin in chronic cyanide poisoning, *J. Toxicol. Clin. Exp.*, **8** (1988) 35–38.

32. J. E. Cottrell, P. Casthely, J. D. Brodie, K. Patel, A. Klein, H. Turndorf, Prevention of nitroprusside-induced cyanide toxicity with hydroxocobalamin, *New Engl. J. Med.*, **298** (1978) 809–811.

33. A. H. Hall, K. Kulig, B. Rumack, Suspected cyanide poisoning in smoke inhalation: complications of sodium nitrite therapy, *J. Toxicol. Clin. Exp.*, **9** (1989) 3–9.

34. L. MacLennan, N. Moiemen, Management of cyanide toxicity in patients with burns, *Burns*, **41** (2015) 18–24.

35. L. Nguyen, A. Afshari, S. A. Kahn, S. McGrane, B. Summitt, Utility and outcomes of hydroxocobalamin use in smoke inhalation patients, *Burns*, **43** (2017) 107–113.

36. A. H. Gray, J. Wright, V. Goodey, L. Bruce, *Injectable Drugs Guide*, Pharmaceutical Press, 2010.

37. R. Miller, B. Katzung, In *Basic and Clinical Pharmacology*, ed. B. G. Katzung, Appletion and Lange, USA (1989) pp. 323–333.

38. D. Dodd, M. Johnson, The organic compounds of cobalt (III), *J. Organomet. Chem.*, **52** (1973) 1–232.

39. R. H. Abeles, D. Dolphin, The vitamin B_{12} coenzyme, *Acc. Chem. Res.*, **9** (1976) 114–120.

Chapter 6

Recent Trends

6.1 Introduction

Over recent years, advances in functional cobalamin (Cbl) derivatives for biological and medicinal applications have received increasing attention [1–3]. This trend is probably inspired by the metabolic importance of Cbls and their unique properties, functions and reactivity in biological systems. Earlier developments and achievements have already been briefly reviewed [4, 5], but recent important developments have significantly expanded the knowledge horizon and are thus worth mentioning. One of the most important current practical applications of corrinoids deals with cyanide detoxification and detection [6, 7]. For this purpose, aquacobalamin and related corrinoids are usually applied. These molecules are nontoxic; they bind cyanide with a remarkable affinity and selectivity and represent naturally occurring chromophores. Highlights of recent progress in the field of vitamin B_{12} derivatives for medical uses with an overview on the following are explored: vitamin B_{12} for cyanide detection and detoxification, antivitamins B_{12} for diagnosis and therapy, the use of vitamin B_{12} conjugates and corrinoids as activators of soluble guanylyl cyclase, among others.

Molecular Modelling of Vitamin B_{12} and Its Analogues
Penny Poomani Govender, Francis Opoku, Olaide Olalekan Wahab, and Ephraim Muriithi Kiarii
Copyright © 2022 Jenny Stanford Publishing Pte. Ltd.
ISBN 978-981-4877-58-9 (Hardcover), 978-1-003-21339-0 (eBook)
www.jennystanford.com

6.2 Vitamin B_{12} for Cyanide Detection and Detoxification

Aquacorrinoids represent probably the most promising reagents for cyanide detoxification and detection [6]. This behaviour is based on the remarkably high affinity of cyanide to the CoIII centre of corrinoids [8]. For aquaCbl (H_2OCbl), the binding constant of cyanide equals 10^{14} M^{-1} [8–10], explaining its ideal qualification as a cyanide scavenger. Taking advantage of these properties, Mushett et al. [11] introduced H_2OCbl in 1952 as a favourable antidote for treating cyanide intoxications in mice.

These results were supported by other pioneering studies [12, 13], and H_2OCbl is nowadays administered as one of the most effective antidotes in prehospital intervention [14–16]. The scavenging product, natural B_{12}, is nontoxic and stored in the liver, used further as a provitamin or renally excreted. Therefore, the antidote is tolerated at high doses by humans and shows no interference with tissue oxygenation. However, its application leads to some red-colouring effect, which causes interferences with standard laboratory tests for bilirubin, blood glucose and creatinine [17].

In 1964, Evans suggested aquahydroxycobinamide as a potential alternative [18], since it shows a higher potency as a cyanide scavenger in animal models compared to aquaCbl [18–22]. In 2008, Zelder applied for the first time B_{12} for the quantification of cyanide [23]. Detection is based on the formation of the violet-coloured dicyano–B_{12} complex, with an absorption maximum of the g-band at B 580 nm. In 2009, Männel–Croise and Zelder started a program to study the excellent sensing properties of 'incomplete' corrinoids in more detail. In fact, they demonstrated that the binding of cyanide is controlled by the stereochemistry at the metal centre (a- or b-site) and the nature of the side chains located at the periphery of the macrocycle [24, 25]. The colour of corrinoids changes from orange to violet during cyanide binding, and concentrations as low as 10 mM are detectable by the naked eye. This value is close to the acceptable level of cyanide in drinking water (1.9 mM), as suggested by the World Health Organization (WHO) [26].

6.3 Vitamin B$_{12}$ for Diagnosis and Therapy

Since Paul Ehrlich, who won the Nobel Prize for Medicine in 1908, suggested the concept of the 'magic bullet', a drug which selectively destroys diseased cells but is not harmful to healthy cells [27], a great deal of research has attempted to reach that goal, for instance for the treatment of cancer. In the field of tumour physiology, a crucial step forward was achieved with the discovery of the enhanced permeability and retention (EPR) effect. The first examples deriving from such strategy were described in 1980 with the development of ligand-conjugated liposomes. Since then, many researchers and companies worked on the design of even more efficient drug delivery by active targeting [28–31].

A broad range of ligands have been used for targeted nanocarriers and belong to the families of small molecules, carbohydrates, peptides, proteins or antibodies. Among the small molecules, molecular ligands are often readily available, inexpensive, easy to handle, easy to be chemically modified and easy to be characterised. Among biologically active small molecules, vitamins such as folic acid (FA; vitamin B$_9$) [32, 33], and biotin (vitamin B$_7$) [34] are widely employed for the targeting of cancer cells. Indeed, FA binds with low affinity to the reduced folate carrier virtually present in all cells. Cbl (vitamin B$_{12}$), known to promote the intestinal adsorption of associated molecules, was recently employed for the development of an oral delivery system of insulin in order to bypass subcutaneous administration drawbacks [35].

6.3.1 Diabetes Mellitus

Diabetes mellitus is a disorder of glucose regulation characterised by the accumulation of glucose in the blood [36–38]. In 2013, 382 million people throughout the world suffered from diabetes, and this number is estimated to be 592 million by 2035 [39]. Insulin therapy is essential in the treatment of patients with insulin-dependent diabetes (type 1) and for many patients with non-insulin-dependent diabetes (type 2) [38, 40]. Nanoparticles have been attached to vitamin B$_{12}$ and other polysaccharides in the design of targeted nanoparticles. In the case of dextran, its amidation with succinic acid followed by the amidation reaction with aminoalkyl vitamin B_{12} derivatives assisted by the N-(3-dimethylaminopropyl)-N'-ethylcarbodiimide/N-hydroxysuccinimide (EDC/NHS) resulted, after nanoparticle formulation including insulin entrapment, in dextran–vitamin B_{12} nanoparticles. Amidation (dextran + succinic anhydride) and carbodiimide (vitamin B_{12}–NH_2 + dextran–COOH/ EDC/NHS) which is pathology/target diabetes is incorporated in insulin [41]. The oral delivery of peptide/protein drugs still represents a major challenge due to their poor intrinsic permeability across the intestinal epithelium and the rapid degradation in the gastrointestinal tract. Insulin is being used for decades for the treatment of diabetes, but the molecule does not immediately reach the liver after subcutaneous administration. During the past few decades, several delivery mechanisms have been proposed for effective oral delivery of insulin, including liposomes and polymeric nanocapsules [42]. Chalasani and coworkers designed a dextran-based nanocarrier system decorated with vitamin B_{12} [41], a molecule with confirmed ability to promote the intestine uptake of pharmaceuticals [43].The reported results demonstrated the efficacy of vitamin B_{12} as a targeting moiety for intestinal delivery; however, the supremacy of these delivery systems compared to those clinically employed for insulin delivery needs to be proven.

6.3.2 Cardiovascular Disease

In the early 1990s, elevated blood concentrations of the amino acid homocysteine were associated with increased risk of cardiovascular disease. Supplementation with FA, vitamin B_{12} and vitamin B_6 can lower homocysteine blood concentrations, and therefore, randomised controlled trials (RCTs) using high amounts of FA, either single or in combination with vitamin B_{12} and vitamin B_6, were initiated [44]. These studies followed the hypothesis that large amounts of FA would be effective in reducing elevated homocysteine concentrations (used as an intermediate endpoint) and therefore also reduce the risk of coronary heart disease or stroke [44]. Doses in these trials ranged from 0.8 to 5 mg FA daily, 400–1000 mg vitamin B_{12} and 25–50 mg vitamin B_6; median follow-up periods were between 2 and 7.3 years. One trial in renal patients even used higher vitamin doses (40 mg FA, 2 mg vitamin B_{12} and 100 mg vitamin B_6). Recently, a meta-analysis of eight trials involving about 37,000 patients has been reported in which it was obvious that supplementation with these vitamins neither reduced cardiovascular morbidity or mortality nor total mortality [44].

6.3.3 Epilepsy

"Epilepsy" is a term applied to a group of chronic brain disorders characterised by epileptic seizures. Epilepsy may arise from a variety of different neurological conditions and via many different pathophysiological mechanisms. Some patients have seizures which are often easy to treat, for instance as part of an age-dependent syndrome, while in others the seizures may be therapy-resistant associated with neurologic disabilities. There are about 50 million individuals with epilepsy in the world, and so epilepsy is an important health issue. Infrequent vitamin B disorders may induce epilepsy. Epileptic disorders during the first year of life have a variety of clinical pictures and outcomes. A few of these disorders of infancy are related to the cofactor function of B vitamins. B vitamins play an important role in normal brain function. Inborn errors of metabolism may occasionally affect vitamin B function in the central nervous system. Data on a few hundred cases have been published and are of special interest. Vitamin deficiencies due to malnutrition may sometimes cause brain disorders and seizures.

Vitamin B_{12} is essential for DNA synthesis, in collaboration with folate. Deficiency of vitamin B_{12} is not uncommon among adults, especially the elderly. Haematological and neurological symptoms and signs are the most prominent findings. Inborn errors of Cbl metabolism are rare: Cbl C/D deficiency impairs the synthesis of methyl or adenosylcobalamin (AdoCbl) and can give rise to combined homocystinuria and methylmalonic aciduria, causing severe neurologic symptoms and epilepsy. Therapy with hydroxycobalamin and betaine is rarely successful. Infantile vitamin B_{12} deficiency occurs in babies who are born with a limited hepatic reserve of vitamin B_{12}. The content of vitamin B_{12} in breast milk is important to maintain adequate supplies. Infants of vegetarian mothers or mothers with unrecognised pernicious anaemia may, therefore, develop vitamin B_{12} deficiency. Vitamin B_{12} deficiency may have detrimental neurological effects such as psychomotor

56 | Recent Trends

retardation and epilepsy. Vitamin B_{12} is important for normal brain function.

6.3.4 Cancer

Vitamins are the vital nutrients required for normal cell growth and survival. Especially cancer cells, which have a high metabolic rate, rapid cell division and growth, require a larger amount of vitamins, explaining the higher expression of vitamin receptors on the surface of tumour cells [34]. Imaging unit with vitamins may be a valuable strategy to deliver a specific drug at higher doses to cancer cells. Among the different vitamins, FA, biotin, riboflavin and vitamin B_{12} are essentially required for cancer cell division and are, therefore, used as cancer-targeting units for the selective delivery of anticancer drugs. MiáJeon et al. [45] used biotin as a cancer-targeting unit for the development of glutathione (GSH)-activated theranostic agents 3–6 bearing different drugs and imaging units conjugated through the self-immolative S–S unit. Vineberg et al. [46] also used biotin to develop the dual-warhead theranostics 7a and 7b, which carry two drugs, camptothecin (CPT) and a taxoid, linked with –S–S– linkers on the tripod splitter 1,3,5-triazine. Kennedy et al. [47] studied the conjugation of a suitable drug and reported meta-analysis, which included 18 case-control studies, and nine vitamin B intake or vitamin blood concentrations have also been related to various cancers. The cancer types which have been best investigated with respect to FA are colon cancer and colorectal cancer. Convincing evidence from observational studies led to the initiation of RCTs with FA in colorectal adenomas [47]. However, similar to cardiovascular disease, there seems to be a discrepancy between the observational epidemiological studies, which reported in the majority an inverse association of folate and cancer risk, and the effect of FA supplementation in the RCTs, which reported no effect of FA on recurrence of colorectal adenoma risk [47].

6.3.5 Dementia

Age-related cognitive changes include mild memory loss, cognitive impairment and dementia. There is a substantial degree of overlap among these conditions, and although there are a number of widely accepted tests of cognitive performance, it has to be acknowledged that the different tests measure different domains of cognitive function and complicate direct comparisons of studies. In observational studies, a low folate status and elevated homocysteine levels were associated with poor cognitive test performance, as summarised by Raman et al. [48]. These authors also stated that it is large. The addition of vitamin B_{12} to FA or the supplementation with vitamin B_{12} alone does not seem to alter either the results or the conclusion of the RCTs by Malouf and Grimley Evans [49, 50].

6.3.6 Renal Disease

End-stage renal disease (ESRD) is associated with an age-adjusted mortality rate of 3.5–4 times that in the general population, mainly because of increased cardiovascular mortality [51]. Among other factors, nutritional status is believed to play a key role in determining survival [52]. The components of nutritional status in ESRD patients which may give cause for concern are the protein and amino acid metabolism and vitamin status. Vitamin supplementation with water-soluble vitamins is widely used in ESRD patients to counteract the restricted intake, increased losses and altered metabolism. The percentage of patients receiving supplements of water-soluble vitamins varies widely [53]. The first guidelines on vitamin use in ESRD were published in 2007 [54]. Although observational studies have shown that vitamin supplementation may reduce mortality in ESRD patients [55], the results of the first RCT with vitamin B intervention in patients with advanced chronic kidney disease and ESRD did not confirm this observation [56].

As the kidney has a major role in vitamin B metabolism, it is plausible that chronic kidney disease may affect the vitamin status to a clinically significant extent (Table 6.1). This holds especially true in ESRD, when the dialysis process may cause additionally vitamin losses, as reported by Heinz et al. [57]. Although vitamin supplementation among patients with ESRD is widely practised, the scientific evidence for doing so was, until recently, very vague. Contrary to common beliefs, supplementation with B vitamins in patients with either chronic kidney disease or ESRD affected neither cardiovascular morbidity and mortality nor total mortality [44, 57, 58].

Table 6.1   Overview of evidence for the risk estimate of several clinical endpoints from RCTs with B vitamins

Disease/Outcome	Vitamin	Proposed mechanisms	Level of evidence	Ref.
Mortality	FA, vitamin B_{12}, vitamin B_6	Homocysteine reduction	Meta-analysis of RCTs: no evidence of reduced risk	[44]
Coronary heart disease	FA cobalamin (vitamin B_{12}) Pyridoxine (vitamin B_6)	Homocysteine reduction Reduction of VLDL and LDL cholesterol, increase in HDL cholesterol	Meta-analysis of RCTs: supplementation in patients do not affect the risk of a recurrent event Meta-analysis shows risk reduction in secondary prevention at high doses	[44, 59]
Stroke	Folate/FA cobalamin (vitamin B_{12}) Pyridoxine (vitamin B_6)	Homocysteine reduction	Meta-analysis of RCTs: supplementation in patients do not affect the risk of a recurrent event	[44]
Cognitive decline	FA Vitamin B_{12}	Methylation, homocysteine reduction	RCTs with FA did not improve cognitive function RCTs with vitamin B_{12} did not improve cognitive function	[49, 50]

HDL, high-density lipoprotein; LDL, low-density lipoprotein; VLDL, very-low-density lipoprotein

6.4 Antivitamins B$_{12}$

Antivitamins represent a broad class of compounds which counteract the essential effects of vitamins. The symptoms triggered by antinutritional factors resemble those of vitamin deficiencies but can be successfully reversed by treating patients with the intact vitamin. Despite being undesirable for healthy organisms, the toxicities of these compounds present considerable interest for biological and medicinal purposes. Indeed, antivitamins played fundamental roles in the development of pioneering antibiotic and antiproliferative drugs, such as prontosil and aminopterin. Their development and optimisation were made possible by the study, throughout the 20th century, of the vitamins' and antivitamins' functions in metabolic processes. However, even with this thorough knowledge, commercialised antivitamin-based drugs are still nowadays limited to antagonists of vitamins B$_9$ and K. The antivitamin field thus still needs to be explored more intensely, in view of the outstanding therapeutic success exhibited by several antivitamin-based medicines. Antivitamins counteract the essential effects of vitamins, for example by inhibiting vitamin-dependent enzymes [2, 60]. Definitions, classifications and efforts towards the development of antivitamins B$_{12}$ have been recently reviewed [2, 60]. This book highlights two recent examples, one report by Zhou et al. [61, 62] and Mutti et al. [63, 64].

Antivitamins entertain a pairwise functional relationship with respect to their physiological effects. Classifying vitamin–antivitamin pairs on the basis of their opposing metabolic roles in humans and other mammals has been used as the basis of classification. Besides these criteria, broader considerations may, for example, include a wider range of organisms [2, 65]. Antivitamins, structured similarly to their vitamin counterparts and, thus, primarily acting as competitive multifunctional inhibitors, are classified here as type I antivitamins. Others, the type II antivitamins, have more diverse structures and physiological roles, and they may, mostly, act indirectly. They may reduce the effective cellular activity of vitamins, for example, by direct destruction of the vitamin, by inhibiting the formation of active vitamin forms or by inhibiting cellular access of the vitamin [66]. Zelder et al. [2] studied a 'biochemical' classification of antivitamins as inhibitors or as modifiers. Antivitamins of either type may be helpful therapeutics counteracting particular vitamins, in case the activity of the latter needs to be reduced to prevent serious health problems. For example, compounds broadly classified as type II antivitamins K, such as the coumarines and acenocoumarol, are used in therapies preventing excessive blood clotting and thrombosis [67, 68].

Antivitamin-type compounds may develop a beneficial effect by interfering selectively with the metabolism of bacterial or fungal pathogens, in addition to being explored as anticancerous agents [69]. Antifolates, such as methotrexate, have been applied along these lines as antibiotics inhibiting folate-dependent enzymatic processes in bacteria [70, 71].

By taking into account the structural requirements of vitamins for their uptake, for intra- and intercellular transport and for their physiological modes of action [72], corresponding antivitamins of type I may be designed rationally when structured very similarly and lacking the specific metabolic reactivity of the reference vitamin [64]. Vitamin B_{12} deficiency causes widespread health problems [73], whereas 'overdoses' of vitamin B_{12} appear to have no toxic effects. Now, how could studies about antivitamins B_{12} contribute to this topic? Indeed, a growing number of suspected contributions of vitamin B_{12} deficiency to pathological phenomena have come into focus, such as degenerative diseases of the central and peripheral nervous systems. Therefore, studies of vitamin B_{12} deficiency in laboratory animals have been helpful. In fact, to induce and investigate effects of vitamin B_{12} deficiency efficiently, deep surgery ('total' gastrectomy) has been routinely practiced on laboratory mice [74, 75], with corresponding ethical implications and with serious physiological interferences unrelated to the specific vitamin B_{12}–related questions [76]. Alternative means for inducing vitamin B_{12} deficiency in animals have become highly desirable. Indeed, application of metabolically 'locked' analogues of vitamin B_{12} could be a 'humane' way of inducing 'functional' vitamin B_{12} deficiency [64].

Metabolically inert Cbls with molecular structures similar to CNCbl or AdoCbl could be taken up in mammals like vitamin B_{12} without subsequent conversion into proper vitamin B_{12} cofactors. Such 'dummy' vitamin B_{12} analogues should, thus, cause 'functional' vitamin B_{12} deficiency. Therefore, metabolically inert Cbls have excellent potential as (broadly effective) antivitamins B_{12} and are classified here (more specifically) as 'type I' antivitamins B_{12}. Remarkably, the historically used anaesthetic 'laughing gas' (N_2O) would be a 'type II antivitamin B_{12}', as it interferes effectively with MetH by oxidising the reduced vitamin B_{12} form Cbl(I) [77].

Antivitamins B_{12} are to be considered poisons for humans, and a direct diagnostic or therapeutic benefit from their use is not foreseeable at present. However, studies of the effects of antivitamins B_{12} with healthy animals are expected, first of all, to help recognise hallmarks of 'functional vitamin B_{12} deficiency'. Due to a deficit of the cofactors of the two vitamin B_{12}–dependent enzymes, these are the accumulation of homocysteine and of methylmalonic acid [78] and a corresponding lack of methionine and of free folate [79]. Among further downstream consequences of an inactive methyltransferase MetH, an insufficient supply with S-adenosyl-methionine would be assumed to result and, thus, for example, deranged epigenomics would be expected [76], due to a lack of proper DNA methylation [80]. It is, therefore, of interest to better relate the expected metabolic changes with puzzling consequences of vitamin B_{12} deficiency, which often still lack a sound physiological or metabolic rationalisation. Among these are the degenerative brain and nerve diseases in humans [81], noted changes in the availability of important growth factors correlating with vitamin B_{12} deficiency, altered profiles of cellular proliferation [82], impaired reproduction [83] and impaired development [74, 84].

Investigations with animals of the pathological effects of antivitamins B_{12} may also lead to the discovery of yet unknown roles of Cbls. Among these are, potentially, vitamin B_{12}–dependent mechanisms which exploit the behaviour of Cbls as high-affinity ligands of regulatory biomacromolecules (Fig. 6.1), thus representing the largely elusive 'noncanonical' roles of Cbls in mammals [85]. The unique 3D structures of Cbls have been exploited by nature for regulatory roles using RNA-based riboswitches [86], which were discovered in studies of what became known as the BtuB B_{12} riboswitch of *Escherichia coli* [87]. This vitamin B_{12} riboswitch appears to recognise and to bind Cbls and related 'complete' corrinoids in their base-on structures and, yet, to display a remarkable structural tolerance for the axial ligands at the corrin-bound Co III centre [88].

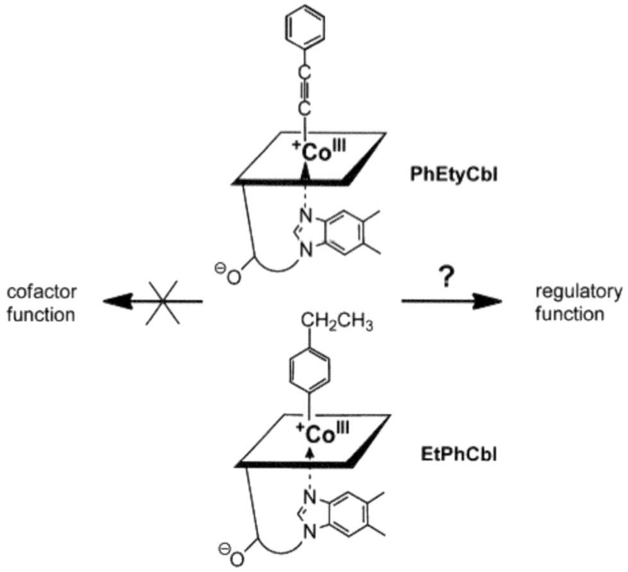

Figure 6.1 EtPhCbl and PhEtyCbl are examples of aryl- and alkynyl-Cbls, respectively, two classes of (potentially) effective antivitamins B_{12}. These 'B$_{12}$ dummies' induce 'functional vitamin B_{12} deficiency' by lacking (blocking) cofactor activity of Cbls (as shown in mice) and may (still) function in regulatory roles of Cbls in mammals [60].

6.5 Vitamin B_{12} in Biological Systems

Nature has always been the ultimate source of inspiration for scientists working across all disciplines. This statement certainly applies to catalysis, where continuous effort has been invested in mimicking and improving the function and effectiveness of enzymes. To this end, new synthetic catalysts have been developed and exploited to facilitate more efficient and selective transformations of organic compounds. However, many of these catalysts are poor replicas of naturally occurring enzymes, compromised by low stability or selectivity, high catalyst loading or toxicity.

Nicholas Lunin studied the effect of salt content on mice maintained on artificial food. The mice, however, could not survive for very long, irrespective of the salt content of the food. Lunin concluded that natural food such as milk must, therefore, contain, besides these known principal ingredients, small quantities of unknown substances essential to life [89]. First isolated by Folkers and Smith in 1948 [90, 91], vitamin B_{12} has been known as a cofactor for enzymes that catalyse a range of biological processes, including isomerisation, methyltransferase and dehalogenation [92].

Cbl (1) as a cofactor for methylcobalamin (MeCbl)-dependent and AdoCbl-dependent enzymes plays a key role in biological processes, including DNA synthesis and regulation, nervous system function, red blood cell formation, etc. Enzymatic reactions, such as isomerisation, dehalogenation and methyl transfer, rely on the formation and cleavage of the Co–C bond. Because it is a natural, nontoxic, environmentally benign cobalt complex, Cbl (1) has been successfully utilised in organic synthesis as a catalyst for Co-mediated reactions. Microbes which possess vitamin B_{12}–dependent reductive dehalogenases can remove halogen substituents from organic halides. Over the years, these reactions have attracted a lot of attention due to their potential application in remediation of persistent polyhalogenated pollutants among other vitamin B_{12}–catalysed reactions [93].

The coupling of therapeutic agents to vitamin B_{12} (1) has been a major goal for many researchers due to vitamin B_{12} possessing a specific uptake pathway [94]. Furthermore, the chemical synthesis of coenzymes (adenosylcobamide and methylcobamide) from vitamin B_{12} is important as they work in unison with enzymes to catalyse rearrangement and methyl transfer reactions, respectively [95]. A Cbl derivative, cobinamide, is used for cyanide detection in solution and in blood and has also been utilised in the separation of different Cbl-binding proteins, such as transcobalamin (TC), intrinsic factor (IF) and haptocorrin (HC), within various excreted substances from fish [96] and mammals [97].

It can also be employed in soluble guanylyl cyclase (sGC) regulation, activating the enzyme through the catalytic domain, whereas other activating agents target the regulatory domain [98]. Vitamin B_{12} derivatives have also been studied as catalysts in dehalogenation reactions [99]. From an environmental point of view, this method shows promising results for converting pollutants such as 1,1-bis(4-chlorophenyl)-2,2,2-trichloroethane (DDT) into less harmful 1,1-bis(4-chlorophenyl)-2,2-dichloroethane (DDD) [99]. A similar type of reaction has also been utilised in the detoxification of inorganic arsenic [100].

Vitamin B_{12} cofactors play important roles in the metabolism of microorganisms, animals and humans. Microorganisms are the only natural sources of vitamin B_{12} derivatives [85], and the latter are vitamins for other vitamin B_{12}–requiring organisms. Some vitamin B_{12}–dependent enzymes catalyse complex isomerisation reactions, such as methylmalonyl-CoA mutase. Vitamin B_{12} is required to induce enzymatic radical reactions. Another group of widely relevant enzymes catalyses the transfer of methyl groups, such as methionine synthase, which uses MeCbl as a cofactor. This chapter covers the structure and reactivity of vitamin B_{12} derivatives and structural aspects of their interactions with proteins and nucleotides, which are crucial for the efficient catalysis by the important vitamin B_{12}–dependent enzymes and for achieving and regulating uptake and transport of B_{12} derivatives.

References

1. F. H. Zelder, C. Männel-Croisé, Recent advances in the colorimetric detection of cyanide, *CHIMIA Int. J. Chem.*, **63** (2009) 58–62.

2. F. Zelder, M. Sonnay, L. Prieto, Antivitamins for medicinal applications, *ChemBioChem*, **16** (2015) 1264–1278.

3. B. Szyszko, L. Latos-Grażyński, Core chemistry and skeletal rearrangements of porphyrinoids and metalloporphyrinoids, *Chem. Soc. Rev.*, **44** (2015) 3588–3616.

4. K. M. Kadish, K. M. Smith, *Handbook of Porphyrin Science: With Applications to Chemistry, Physics, Materials Science, Engineering, Biology and Medicine*, World Scientific, 2013.

5. W. Friedrich, *Vitamin B_{12} und verwandte Corrinoide*, Thieme, 1975.

6. G. Shepherd, L. I. Velez, Role of hydroxocobalamin in acute cyanide poisoning, *Ann. Pharmacother.*, **42** (2008) 661–669.

7. J. E. Cottrell, P. Casthely, J. D. Brodie, K. Patel, A. Klein, H. Turndorf, Prevention of nitroprusside-induced cyanide toxicity with hydroxocobalamin, *New Engl. J. Med.*, **298** (1978) 809–811.

8. G. Schrauzer, *Inorganic Chemistry of Vitamin B_{12}*, Academic Press, New York, USA, 1972.

9. S. M. Chemaly, Cobalamins and the spectrochemical series, *Dalton Trans.*, (2008) 5766–5773.

References

10. B. Kräutler, B. T. Golding, D. Arigoni, *Vitamin B_{12} and B_{12}-Proteins*, John Wiley & Sons, 2008.

11. C. W. Mushett, K. L. Kelley, G. E. Boxer, J. C. Rickards, Antidotal efficacy of vitamin B_{12a} (hydroxo-cobalamin) in experimental cyanide poisoning, *Proc. Soc. Exp. Biol. Med.*, **81** (1952) 234–237.

12. F. Zelder, Recent trends in the development of vitamin B_{12} derivatives for medicinal applications, *Chem. Commun.*, **51** (2015) 14004–14017.

13. J. Delga, J. Mizoule, B. Veverka, R. Bon, Research on the treatment of hydrocyanic intoxication with hydroxy-cobalamine, *Ann. Pharm. Fr.*, **19** (1961) 740–752.

14. J.-L. Fortin, J.-P. Giocanti, M. Ruttimann, J.-J. Kowalski, Prehospital administration of hydroxocobalamin for smoke inhalation-associated cyanide poisoning: 8 years of experience in the Paris Fire Brigade, *Clin. Toxicol.*, **44** (2006) 37–44.

15. S. W. Borron, F. J. Baud, P. Barriot, M. Imbert, C. Bismuth, Prospective study of hydroxocobalamin for acute cyanide poisoning in smoke inhalation, *Ann. Emergency Med.*, **49** (2007) 794–801.e792.

16. J. Fortin, T. Desmettre, J. Peureux, J. Giocanti, P. Luporsi, G. Capellier, fire smoke inhalation and cardiac disorders–efficacy of hydroxocobalamin: final results, in *Clin. Toxicol.*, Informa Healthcare 52 Vanderbilt Ave, New York, NY 10017 USA, 2012, pp. 301–301.

17. N. Beckerman, S. M. Leikin, R. Aitchinson, M. Yen, B. K. Wills, Laboratory interferences with the newer cyanide antidote: hydroxocobalamin, in *Semin. Diagn. Pathol.*, Elsevier, 2009, pp. 49–52.

18. C. L. Evans, Cobalt compounds as antidotes for hydrocyanic acid, *Br. J. Pharmacol.*, **23** (1964) 455–475.

19. K. E. Broderick, P. Potluri, S. Zhuang, I. E. Scheffler, V. S. Sharma, R. B. Pilz, G. R. Boss, Cyanide detoxification by the cobalamin precursor cobinamide, *Exp. Biol. Med.*, **231** (2006) 641–649.

20. M. Brenner, S. B. Mahon, J. Lee, J. Kim, D. Mukai, S. Goodman, K. A. Kreuter, R. Ahdout, O. Mohammad, V. S. Sharma, Comparison of cobinamide to hydroxocobalamin in reversing cyanide physiologic effects in rabbits using diffuse optical spectroscopy monitoring, *J. Biomed. Opt.*, **15** (2010) 017001.

21. A. Chan, M. Balasubramanian, W. Blackledge, O. M. Mohammad, L. Alvarez, G. R. Boss, T. D. Bigby, Cobinamide is superior to other treatments in a mouse model of cyanide poisoning, *Clin. Toxicol.*, **48** (2010) 709–717.

22. V. S. Bebarta, D. A. Tanen, S. Boudreau, M. Castaneda, L. A. Zarzabal, T. Vargas, G. R. Boss, Intravenous cobinamide versus hydroxocobalamin for acute treatment of severe cyanide poisoning in a swine (Sus scrofa) model, *Ann. Emergency Med.*, **64** (2014) 612–619.

23. F. H. Zelder, Specific colorimetric detection of cyanide triggered by a conformational switch in vitamin B_{12}, *Inorg. Chem.*, **47** (2008) 1264–1266.

24. B. Aebli, C. Männel-Croisé, F. Zelder, Controlling binding dynamics of corrin-based chemosensors for cyanide, *Inorg. Chem.*, **53** (2014) 2516–2520.

25. C. Männel-Croisé, F. Zelder, Side chains of cobalt corrinoids control the sensitivity and selectivity in the colorimetric detection of cyanide, *Inorg. Chem.*, **48** (2009) 1272–1274.

26. T. Thompson, J. Fawell, S. Kunikane, D. Jackson, S. Appleyard, P. Callan, J. Bartram, P. Kingston, *Chemical Safety of Drinking Water: Assessing Priorities for Risk Management*, World Health Organization, 2007.

27. K. Strebhardt, A. Ullrich, Paul Ehrlich's magic bullet concept: 100 years of progress, *Nat. Rev. Cancer*, **8** (2008) 473 480.

28. M. R. Dreher, W. Liu, C. R. Michelich, M. W. Dewhirst, F. Yuan, A. Chilkoti, Tumor vascular permeability, accumulation, and penetration of macromolecular drug carriers, *J. Natl. Cancer Inst.*, **98** (2006) 335–344.

29. A. K. Iyer, G. Khaled, J. Fang, H. Maeda, Exploiting the enhanced permeability and retention effect for tumor targeting, *Drug Discovery Today*, **11** (2006) 812–818.

30. M. Elsabahy, K. L. Wooley, Design of polymeric nanoparticles for biomedical delivery applications, *Chem. Soc. Rev.*, **41** (2012) 2545–2561.

31. E. Gullotti, Y. Yeo, Extracellularly activated nanocarriers: a new paradigm of tumor targeted drug delivery, *Mol. Pharm.*, **6** (2009) 1041–1051.

32. P. S. Low, W. A. Henne, D. D. Doorneweerd, Discovery and development of folic-acid-based receptor targeting for imaging and therapy of cancer and inflammatory diseases, *Acc. Chem. Res.*, **41** (2007) 120–129.

33. Y. Lu, E. Sega, C. P. Leamon, P. S. Low, Folate receptor-targeted immunotherapy of cancer: mechanism and therapeutic potential, *Adv. Drug Del. Rev.*, **56** (2004) 1161–1176.

34. G. Russell-Jones, K. McTavish, J. McEwan, J. Rice, D. Nowotnik, Vitamin-mediated targeting as a potential mechanism to increase drug uptake by tumours, *J. Inorg. Biochem.*, **98** (2004) 1625–1633.

35. G. Russell-Jones, S. Westwood, A. Habberfield, Vitamin B_{12} mediated oral delivery systems for granulocyte-colony stimulating factor and erythropoietin, *Bioconjugate Chem.*, **6** (1995) 459–465.

36. M. A. Atkinson, G. S. Eisenbarth, A. W. Michels, Type 1 diabetes, *Lancet*, **383** (2014) 69–82.

37. M. A. Atkinson, G. S. Eisenbarth, Type 1 diabetes: new perspectives on disease pathogenesis and treatment, *Lancet*, **358** (2001) 221–229.

38. M. Stumvoll, B. J. Goldstein, T. W. van Haeften, Type 2 diabetes: principles of pathogenesis and therapy, *Lancet*, **365** (2005) 1333–1346.

39. J. E. Shaw, R. A. Sicree, P. Z. Zimmet, Global estimates of the prevalence of diabetes for 2010 and 2030, *Diabetes Res. Clin. Pract.*, **87** (2010) 4–14.

40. D. R. Owens, B. Zinman, G. B. Bolli, Insulins today and beyond, *Lancet*, **358** (2001) 739–746.

41. K. B. Chalasani, G. J. Russell-Jones, A. K. Jain, P. V. Diwan, S. K. Jain, Effective oral delivery of insulin in animal models using vitamin B_{12}-coated dextran nanoparticles, *J. Controlled Release*, **122** (2007) 141–150.

42. M. Kisel, L. Kulik, I. Tsybovsky, A. Vlasov, M. Vorob'Yov, E. Kholodova, Z. Zabarovskaya, Liposomes with phosphatidylethanol as a carrier for oral delivery of insulin: studies in the rat, *Int. J. Pharm.*, **216** (2001) 105–114.

43. G. Russell-Jones, S. Westwood, P. Farnworth, J. Findlay, H. Burger, Synthesis of LHRH antagonists suitable for oral administration via the vitamin B_{12} uptake system, *Bioconjugate Chem.*, **6** (1995) 34–42.

44. R. Clarke, J. Halsey, S. Lewington, E. Lonn, J. Armitage, J. E. Manson, K. H. Bønaa, J. D. Spence, O. Nygård, R. Jamison, Effects of lowering homocysteine levels with B vitamins on cardiovascular disease, cancer, and cause-specific mortality: meta-analysis of 8 randomized trials involving 37 485 individuals, *Arch. Intern. Med.*, **170** (2010) 1622–1631.

45. H. MiáJeon, H. ThiáLe, T. WooáKim, J. SeungáKim, A biotin-guided fluorescent-peptide drug delivery system for cancer treatment, *Chem. Commun.*, **50** (2014) 7690–7693.

46. J. G. Vineberg, E. S. Zuniga, A. Kamath, Y.-J. Chen, J. D. Seitz, I. Ojima, Design, synthesis, and biological evaluations of tumor-targeting dual-warhead conjugates for a taxoid-camptothecin combination chemotherapy, *J. Med. Chem.*, **57** (2014) 5777–5791.

47. D. A. Kennedy, S. J. Stern, M. Moretti, I. Matok, M. Sarkar, C. Nickel, G. Koren, Folate intake and the risk of colorectal cancer: a systematic review and meta-analysis, *Cancer Epidemiol.*, **35** (2011) 2–10.

48. G. Raman, A. Tatsioni, M. Chung, I. H. Rosenberg, J. Lau, A. H. Lichtenstein, E. M. Balk, Heterogeneity and lack of good quality studies limit association between folate, vitamins B-6 and B-12, and cognitive function, *J. Nutr.*, **137** (2007) 1789–1794.

49. D. S. Wald, A. Kasturiratne, M. Simmonds, Effect of folic acid, with or without other B vitamins, on cognitive decline: meta-analysis of randomized trials, *Am. J. Med.*, **123** (2010) 522–527.

50. S. J. Eussen, L. C. de Groot, L. W. Joosten, R. J. Bloo, R. Clarke, P. M. Ueland, J. Schneede, H. J. Blom, W. H. Hoefnagels, W. A. van Staveren, Effect of oral vitamin B_{12} with or without folic acid on cognitive function in older people with mild vitamin B_{12} deficiency: a randomized, placebo-controlled trial, *Am. J. Clin. Nutr.*, **84** (2006) 361–370.

51. R. N. Foley, P. S. Parfrey, M. J. Sarnak, Epidemiology of cardiovascular disease in chronic renal disease, *J. Am. Soc. Nephrol.*, **9** (1998) S16–23.

52. J. Zimmermann, S. Herrlinger, A. Pruy, T. Metzger, C. Wanner, Inflammation enhances cardiovascular risk and mortality in hemodialysis patients, *Kidney Int.*, **55** (1999) 648–658.

53. R. B. Fissell, J. L. Bragg-Gresham, B. W. Gillespie, D. A. Goodkin, J. Bommer, A. Saito, T. Akiba, F. K. Port, E. W. Young, International variation in vitamin prescription and association with mortality in the Dialysis Outcomes and Practice Patterns Study (DOPPS), *Am. J. Kidney Dis.*, **44** (2004) 293–299.

54. D. Fouque, M. Vennegoor, P. ter Wee, C. Wanner, A. Basci, B. Canaud, P. Haage, K. Konner, J. Kooman, A. Martin-Malo, L. Pedrini, F. Pizzarelli, J. Tattersall, J. Tordoir, R. Vanholder, EBPG guideline on nutrition, *Nephrol. Dial. Transplant.*, **22**(Suppl 2) (2007) ii45–87.

55. U. Domröse, J. Heinz, S. Westphal, C. Luley, K. Neumann, J. Dierkes, Vitamins are associated with survival in patients with end-stage renal disease: a 4-year prospective study, *Clin. Nephrol.*, **67** (2007) 221–229.

56. R. L. Jamison, P. Hartigan, J. S. Kaufman, D. S. Goldfarb, S. R. Warren, P. D. Guarino, J. M. Gaziano, V. A. S. Investigators, Effect of homocysteine lowering on mortality and vascular disease in advanced chronic kidney disease and end-stage renal disease: a randomized controlled trial, *JAMA*, **298** (2007) 1163–1170.

57. J. Heinz, U. Domröse, S. Westphal, C. Luley, K. H. Neumann, J. Dierkes, Washout of water-soluble vitamins and of homocysteine during

haemodialysis: effect of high-flux and low-flux dialyser membranes, *Nephrology*, **13** (2008) 384–389.

58. A. G. Bostom, M. A. Carpenter, J. W. Kusek, A. S. Levey, L. Hunsicker, M. A. Pfeffer, J. Selhub, P. F. Jacques, E. Cole, L. Gravens-Mueller, Homocysteine-lowering and cardiovascular disease outcomes in kidney transplant recipients, *Circulation*, **123** (2011) 1763–1770.

59. E. Bruckert, J. Labreuche, P. Amarenco, Meta-analysis of the effect of nicotinic acid alone or in combination on cardiovascular events and atherosclerosis, *Atherosclerosis*, **210** (2010) 353–361.

60. B. Kräutler, Antivitamins B_{12}-a structure- and reactivity-based concept, *Chem. Eur. J.*, **21** (2015) 11280–11287.

61. K. Zhou, F. Zelder, Vitamin B_{12} mimics having a peptide backbone and tuneable coordination and redox properties, *Angew. Chem. Int. Ed.*, **49** (2010) 5178–5180.

62. K. Zhou, R. M. Oetterli, H. Brandl, F. E. Lyatuu, W. Buckel, F. Zelder, Chemistry and bioactivity of an artificial adenosylpeptide B_{12} cofactor, *ChemBioChem*, **13** (2012) 2052–2055.

63. E. Mutti, M. Ruetz, H. Birn, B. Kräutler, E. Nexo, 4-ethylphenyl-cobalamin impairs tissue uptake of vitamin B_{12} and causes vitamin B_{12} deficiency in mice, *PLoS One*, **8** (2013) e75312.

64. M. Ruetz, C. Gherasim, K. Gruber, S. Fedosov, R. Banerjee, B. Kräutler, Access to organometallic arylcobaltcorrins through radical synthesis: 4-ethylphenylcobalamin, a potential "Antivitamin B_{12}", *Angew. Chem. Int. Ed.*, **52** (2013) 2606–2610.

65. M. T. Croft, M. J. Warren, A. G. Smith, Algae need their vitamins, *Eukaryot. Cell*, **5** (2006) 1175–1183.

66. H. Kläui, Inactivation of vitamins, *Proc. Nutr. Soc.*, **38** (1979) 135–141.

67. J. Hirsh, M. O'Donnell, J. W. Eikelboom, Beyond unfractionated heparin and warfarin, *Circulation*, **116** (2007) 552–560.

68. 8] M. D. Freedman, Warfarin and other "anti"-vitamin K anticoagulants: pharmacodynamics and clinical use, *Am. J. Ther.*, **3** (1996) 771–783.

69. S. Farber, L. K. Diamond, R. D. Mercer, R. F. Sylvester Jr, J. A. Wolff, Temporary remissions in acute leukemia in children produced by folic acid antagonist, 4-aminopteroyl-glutamic acid (aminopterin), *New Engl. J. Med.*, **238** (1948) 787–793.

70. M. P. Pereira, S. O. Kelley, Maximizing the therapeutic window of an antimicrobial drug by imparting mitochondrial sequestration in human cells, *J. Am. Chem. Soc.*, **133** (2011) 3260–3263.

71. A. Bermingham, J. P. Derrick, The folic acid biosynthesis pathway in bacteria: evaluation of potential for antibacterial drug discovery, *Bioessays*, **24** (2002) 637–648.

72. M. Eggersdorfer, D. Laudert, U. Létinois, T. McClymont, J. Medlock, T. Netscher, W. Bonrath, One hundred years of vitamins–a success story of the natural sciences, *Angew. Chem. Int. Ed.*, **51** (2012) 12960–12990.

73. N. E. Allen, Plasma selenium concentration and prostate cancer risk Reply, *Am. J. Clin. Nutr.*, **89** (2009) 1277–1277.

74. G. Scalabrino, M. Peracchi, New insights into the pathophysiology of cobalamin deficiency, *Trends Mol. Med.*, **12** (2006) 247–254.

75. G. Scalabrino, D. Veber, E. Mutti, Experimental and clinical evidence of the role of cytokines and growth factors in the pathogenesis of acquired cobalamin-deficient leukoneuropathy, *Brain Res. Rev.*, **59** (2008) 42–54.

76. J.-L. Guéant, M. Caillerez-Fofou, S. Battaglia-Hsu, J.-M. Alberto, J.-N. Freund, I. Dulluc, C. Adjalla, F. Maury, C. Merle, J.-P. Nicolas, Molecular and cellular effects of vitamin B_{12} in brain, myocardium and liver through its role as co factor of methionine synthase, *Biochimie*, **95** (2013) 1033–1040.

77. J. T. Drummond, R. G. Matthews, Nitrous oxide degradation by cobalamin-dependent methionine synthase: characterization of the reactants and products in the inactivation reaction, *Biochemistry*, **33** (1994) 3732–3741.

78. E. Mutti, V. Magnaghi, D. Veber, A. Faroni, S. Pece, P. P. Di Fiore, G. Scalabrino, Cobalamin deficiency-induced changes of epidermal growth factor (EGF)-receptor expression and EGF levels in rat spinal cord, *Brain Res.*, **1376** (2011) 23–30.

79. E. Reynolds, Vitamin B12, folic acid, and the nervous system, *Lancet Neurol.*, **5** (2006) 949–960.

80. J. Geisel, H. Schorr, M. Bodis, S. Isber, U. Hübner, J.-P. Knapp, R. Obeid, W. Herrmann, The vegetarian lifestyle and DNA methylation, *Clin. Chem. Lab. Med.*, **43** (2005) 1164–1169.

81. G. Scalabrino, The multi-faceted basis of vitamin B_{12} (cobalamin) neurotrophism in adult central nervous system: lessons learned from its deficiency, *Prog. Neurobiol.*, **88** (2009) 203–220.

82. S.-F. Battaglia-Hsu, N. Akchiche, N. Noel, J.-M. Alberto, E. Jeannesson, C. E. Orozco-Barrios, D. Martinez-Fong, J.-L. Daval, J.-L. Guéant, Vitamin B_{12} deficiency reduces proliferation and promotes differentiation of

neuroblastoma cells and up-regulates PP2A, proNGF, and TACE, *Proc. Natl. Acad. Sci.*, **106** (2009) 21930–21935.

83. T. Bito, Y. Matsunaga, Y. Yabuta, T. Kawano, F. Watanabe, Vitamin B_{12} deficiency in Caenorhabditis elegans results in loss of fertility, extended life cycle, and reduced lifespan, *FEBS Open Bio*, **3** (2013) 112–117.

84. G. Scalabrino, D. Veber, G. Tredici, Relationships between cobalamin, epidermal growth factor, and normal prions in the myelin maintenance of central nervous system, *Int. J. Biochem. Cell Biol.*, **55** (2014) 232–241.

85. K. Gruber, B. Puffer, B. Kräutler, Vitamin B_{12}-derivatives-enzyme cofactors and ligands of proteins and nucleic acids, *Chem. Soc. Rev.*, **40** (2011) 4346–4363.

86. R. R. Breaker, Complex riboswitches, *Science*, **319** (2008) 1795–1797.

87. A. Nahvi, J. E. Barrick, R. R. Breaker, Coenzyme B_{12} riboswitches are widespread genetic control elements in prokaryotes, *Nucleic Acids Res.*, **32** (2004) 143–150.

88. S. Gallo, M. Oberhuber, R. K. Sigel, B. Kräutler, The corrin moiety of coenzyme B_{12} is the determinant for switching the btuB riboswitch of *E. coli*, *ChemBioChem*, **9** (2008) 1408–1414.

89. N. Lunin, Ueber die Bedeutung der anorganischen Salze für die Ernährung des Thieres, *Z. Physiol. Chem.*, **5** (1881) 31–39.

90. E. L. Rickes, N. G. Brink, F. R. Koniuszy, T. R. Wood, K. Folkers, Crystalline vitamin B_{12}, *Science (Wash.)*, **107** (1948) 396–397.

91. E. L. Smith, Presence of cobalt in the anti-pernicious anaemia factor, *Nature*, **162** (1948) 144–144.

92. S. Kliegman, K. McNeill, Dechlorination of chloroethylenes by cob (I) alamin and cobalamin model complexes, *Dalton Trans.*, (2008) 4191–4201.

93. M. Giedyk, K. Goliszewska, D. Gryko, Vitamin B_{12} catalysed reactions, *Chem. Soc. Rev.*, **44** (2015) 3391–3404.

94. A. K. Petrus, T. J. Fairchild, R. P. Doyle, Traveling the vitamin B_{12} pathway: oral delivery of protein and peptide drugs, *Angew. Chem. Int. Ed.*, **48** (2009) 1022–1028.

95. K. L. Brown, Chemistry and enzymology of vitamin B_{12}, *Chem. Rev.*, **105** (2005) 2075–2150.

96. E. Greibe, S. Fedosov, E. Nexo, The cobalamin-binding protein in zebrafish is an intermediate between the three cobalamin-binding proteins in human, *PLoS One*, **7** (2012) e35660.

97. C. Männel-Croisé, F. Zelder, Rapid visual detection of blood cyanide, *Anal. Methods*, **4** (2012) 2632–2634.

98. I. Sharina, M. Sobolevsky, M.-F. Doursout, D. Gryko, E. Martin, Cobinamides are novel coactivators of nitric oxide receptor that target soluble guanylyl cyclase catalytic domain, *J. Pharmacol. Exp. Ther.*, **340** (2012) 723–732.

99. M. A. Jabbar, H. Shimakoshi, Y. Hisaeda, Enhanced reactivity of hydrophobic vitamin B_{12} towards the dechlorination of DDT in ionic liquid, *Chem. Commun.*, (2007) 1653–1655.

100. K. Nakamura, Y. Hisaeda, L. Pan, H. Yamauchi, Methyl transfer from a hydrophobic vitamin B_{12} derivative to arsenic trioxide, *J. Organomet. Chem.*, **694** (2009) 916–921.

Chapter 7

Catalysis

7.1 Introduction

For decades, catalysis has remained an indispensable agent of quick positive transformation for life and society. There is always the need for a more accelerated, economic and value-oriented technological development to improve living. The goal of catalysis is the effective optimisation of resources to meet some immediate and future needs. Catalysis is the main driving force for key sectors of the global economy, such as petroleum and energy production, chemicals and polymer manufacturing, the food industry and pollution control. Owing to the increasing world population, the production of numerous beneficial products, including fuels (e.g. gasoline, diesel, heating oil, fuel oil), polymers (e.g. plastics, synthetic rubbers, adhesives, fibres, coatings, foams, fabrics, cables,), foods, drugs and cosmetics needs to be catalysed to meet the expanding needs of mankind. Energy production through water splitting, reduction of automobile emissions and conversion of organic pollutants into harmless form are all catalyst-dependent processes. Catalysis also plays an essential role in living systems. Important biological processes, such as digestion of food substances, metabolism, detoxification and DNA synthesis, are catalysed by specific enzymes in mammals.

Molecular Modelling of Vitamin B$_{12}$ and Its Analogues
Penny Poomani Govender, Francis Opoku, Olaide Olalekan Wahab, and Ephraim Muriithi Kiarii
Copyright © 2022 Jenny Stanford Publishing Pte. Ltd.
ISBN 978-981-4877-58-9 (Hardcover), 978-1-003-21339-0 (eBook)
www.jennystanford.com

7.2 Concept of Catalysis

When the introduction of a small amount of a chemical substance accelerates a spontaneous chemical reaction or allows faster attainment of chemical equilibrium without the substance itself undergoing a permanent chemical change, then the reaction is said to be catalysed. A catalyst is, therefore, defined as a component of a chemical reaction which accelerates the reaction but does not undergo a permanent chemical transformation. It speeds up a chemical reaction by lowering the activation energy of the reaction through the provision of an alternative route which involves a lower energy transition state (Fig. 7.1). A catalyst has no effect on the free energy of a reaction because it is not concerned about the initial and final states of the system. The role of a catalyst is only to increase the reaction speed. This is why a catalyst is not involved in the stoichiometry of a balanced chemical reaction. An inhibitor is the opposite of a catalyst. It decelerates a chemical reaction by increasing its activation energy.

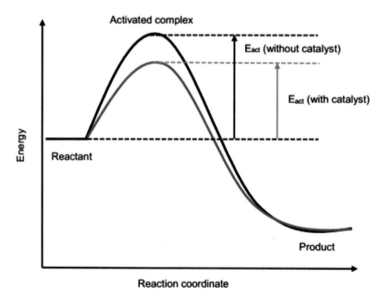

Figure 7.1 Comparison of the activation energies of a catalysed and uncatalysed exothermic process.

7.3 Types of Catalysis

On the basis of the physical state of a catalyst in relation to the target substrate (i.e. reactant), catalysis is broadly classified into two types, homogenous and heterogeneous catalysis.

7.3.1 Homogenous Catalysis

Homogenous catalysis is the type of catalysis in which the catalyst is in the same phase (physical state) as the reactant [1]. That is, the reactant and the catalyst are in one single physical state, which could be gas or liquid. Examples include chlorofluorocarbon (CFC)-catalysed depletion of ozone (O_3), in which both the CFC and O_3 are in the same gaseous phase; nitric oxide–catalysed oxidation of sulphur dioxide; iodine vapour–catalysed decomposition of acetaldehyde; acid-base-catalysed ester and nitrile hydrolysis (liquid phase); and enzyme-catalysed processes (liquid phase). Most vitamin B_{12}–catalysed reactions are homogenous catalytic reactions occurring predominantly in the liquid phase [2].

7.3.2 Heterogeneous Catalysis

In this type of catalysis, the catalyst and the reactant are in different physical states (phases) [3–6]. The catalyst is usually in the solid state, while the reactant can either be in the liquid or the gas phase. Examples of heterogeneous catalytic reactions include platinum- or nickel-catalysed hydrogenation and polymerisation of alkenes; platinum-, palladium- or rhodium-catalysed oxidation of CO gases and reduction of nitrogen oxide gases to reduce pollution; and photocatalytic degradation of organic dyes using powerful oxidising semiconductor or metal oxide catalysts such as TiO_2, ZnO, or WO_3 [7–15]. The reaction sequence illustrated in Fig. 7.2 shows the steps involved in heterogeneous catalytic processes [16–20].

1. Reactant migration to the catalyst surface: This first step of a heterogeneous catalytic reaction involves the movement of reactant molecules (R) from the bulk fluid to the pore mouth on the catalyst surface.

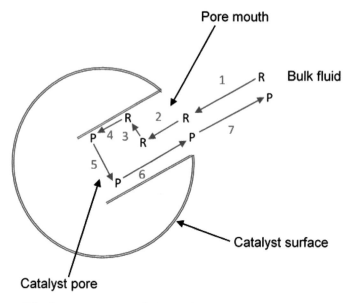

Figure 7.2 Heterogeneous catalytic reaction steps.

2. Reactant diffusion into the catalyst: The reactant molecules diffuse from the pore mouth through the surface pores to the immediate internal portion of the catalyst surface. The rate of diffusion depends on the molecular size and the temperature of the system.
3. Reactant adsorption onto the catalyst surface: This refers to the attachment of the reactant molecules to the immediate inner portion of the catalyst surface through some sort of physical or chemical interactive forces. When the molecules are held onto the surface by weak intermolecular forces, the molecules are said to be physisorbed, and the process is termed 'physisorption' [21, 22]. However, when the surface attachment of the molecules involves the formation of some chemical bonds, the molecules are said to be chemisorbed, and the process is termed 'chemisorption' [21–24].
4. Product formation: The adsorbed molecules undergo chemical transformation through breaking of some chemical bonds and formation of new ones on the catalyst surface to form new

compound(s) (i.e. the product [P]) which is also adsorbed onto the surface.

5. Product desorption: This refers to a detachment of the product formed from the surface of the catalyst into the immediate interior part of the catalyst.
6. Product diffusion to the pore mouth: The product diffuses from the immediate interior part of the catalyst surface through the surface pores to the pore mouth.
7. Product migration to the bulk: The product finally migrates from the pore mouth to the bulk fluid.

The net rate of a heterogeneous catalysed reaction is the rate of the slowest step. In the reaction mechanism highlighted before, if the adsorption (step 3) and reaction (step 4) of the reactant molecules on the catalyst active site are slow compared to their migration (step 1) and diffusion (step 2) from the bulk fluid, the concentration of the reactant molecules in the reaction site is negligibly different from that in the bulk phase. As a result, steps 1 and 2 have no impact on the net rate of the reaction, which implies that the overall rate depends on steps 3 and 4 only. However, if the diffusion (step 2), adsorption (step 3) and reaction (step 4) steps are fast compared to the rate at which the reactant molecules migrate from the bulk to the catalyst (step 1), then the net rate depends only on the reactant migration step. Hence, any slight change in the rate at which the reactant molecules approach the catalyst will alter the overall rate of the reaction.

7.4 Vitamin B$_{12}$: A Unique Natural Organometallic Catalyst

Vitamin B$_{12}$, also known as cobalamin (Cbl), is a versatile natural organometallic complex of interesting catalytic properties. Its versatility lies in its ability to mediate different types of organic reactions of industrial and environmental importance, such as rearrangement, coupling reactions, dehalogenation, transmethylation, cyclopropanation, ring-opening, ring expansion and oxidation [2, 25, 26]. This is due to the ability of the cobalt (Co) atom centre to switch between three different oxidation states in different ligand fields. The different oxidised forms of vitamin B_{12} are B_{12} (III) in which the oxidation state of Co is +3, B_{12} (II) where the oxidation state is +2 and B_{12} (I) in which Co exhibits a +1 oxidation state [2, 27–31]. The last two oxidation states are referred to as reduced (nucleophilic) and super-reduced (super-nucleophilic) states with symbols B_{12r} and B_{12s}, respectively [32, 33]. Naturally, vitamin B_{12} exists in biological systems in the most stable B_{12} (III) form, where the upper axial binding site of the Co–centre (known as the β-position) is coordinated to 5-deoxyadenosyl (Ado) or methyl (CH_3) groups (Fig. 7.3) through the formation of a stable organometallic Co–C bond. Homolytic cleavage of this bond in the 5-deoxyadenosyl derivative (adenosylcobalamin [AdoCbl]) and its heterolytic cleavage in the methyl analogue (methylcobalamin [MeCbl]) give rise to the +2 and +1 states, respectively [2, 32, 33]. Being a form of transition metal complex, the various oxidation states of Cbl exhibit different colours, depending on the oxidation states of the metal ion. B_{12} (II) exhibits a yellow-orange colour, B_{12} (I) appears grey-green, while B_{12} (III), which is the most dominant form, possesses a red colour, and it is therefore called 'red vitamin' [30, 33, 34]. AdoCbl and MeCbl are the two most important natural vitamin B_{12} analogues which act as coenzymes or cofactors for enzymatic reactions such as isomerisation, methyl transfer and reductive dehalogenation in biological systems [2, 30]. They are referred to as coenzymes because they act as facilitators for apoenzyme (apoprotein) catalytic activities in biological systems. An apoenzyme or apoprotein is the protein part of an enzyme which does not contain its characteristic prosthetic group. Other forms of vitamin B_{12} include cyanocobalamin (CNCbl), hydroxocobalamin (HOCbl), aquacobalamin (H_2OCbl) and cyclohexylcobalamin. These forms are converted to the more important biological active derivatives AdoCbl or MeCbl in living systems by replacement of the CN, OH, H_2O or cyclohexyl moieties with 5-deoxyladenosyl or a methyl group.

Vitamin B$_{12}$ | 79

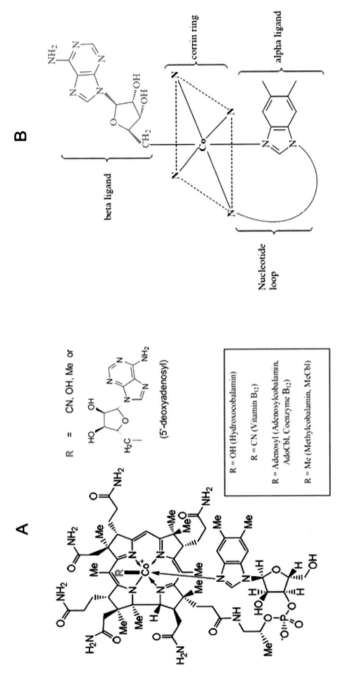

Figure 7.3 Full (A) and simplified (B) illustrations of vitamin B$_{12}$ and its derivatives, where R represents beta ligands [35].

7.5 Catalytic Features of Cobalamins

In the modern-day practice of catalysis, selection of a suitable catalyst for a given chemical process is usually based on some criteria in order to achieve an effective and more environmentally friendly application with minimal cost input. Some of the distinctive features of Cbl derivatives which are responsible for their widespread catalytic application are as follows.

7.5.1 Availability

Cbl can naturally be obtained from serum, liver, organ meat, tissues, shellfish, eggs, fish and cheese and can be produced in the bodies of most mammals. It is predominantly available in the form of CNCbl, which is considered as the most widely manufactured member of the vitamin B_{12} family because of its higher stability, relative ease of crystallisation and purification compared to other members after production through bacterial fermentation. The main Cbls in humans and animals are AdoCbl, MeCbl and HOCbl, where the first two are active coenzyme forms.

7.5.2 Balance between Stability and Reactivity

An important feature of a good catalyst is adequate stability to allow storage over a reasonable period of time. However, high stability is a hindrance to catalytic activity during a reaction, because reactivity is needed in this case. Therefore, an ideal catalyst must possess adequate stability in its free state but instantly become active during a reaction. This requirement is met to a large extent by most vitamin B_{12} derivatives as they quickly become active towards a substrate through a temporary loss of their β-ligand when involved in a chemical reaction. The stability of the Cbl family, particularly the vitamin B_{12} coenzymes, is due to the unprecedented degree of stability of their organometallic Co–C bond, in addition to the central Co–atom obeying the general 18-valence electron rule when the derivatives are in their free state.

7.5.3 Recoverability

As with all catalysts, vitamin B_{12} and its derivatives do not undergo a permanent chemical change when involved in a reaction. They only help to increase the reaction speed and can also serve as a temporary reservoir for ligands or substituent groups to allow the chemical transformation of the substrate. Depending on the reaction type, the ligands may be released as a by-product, as with the case of vitamin B_{12}–catalysed dehalogenation, or situated at a new position in the substrate structure, as with the case of vitamin B_{12}–catalysed rearrangement. The catalysts themselves are recovered at the end of the reaction.

7.5.4 High Activity-to-Dosage Ratio

Cbls possess remarkable catalytic activity, even when used in low dosages. For instance, in a dechlorination study of lindane (an organochlorine pesticide) using CNCbl, AdoCbl, dicyanocobinamide $((CN)_2Cbi)$ and aquacyanocobinamide $((CN)(H_2O)Cbi)$ as catalysts, 800 nanomoles of the pesticide was dechlorinated per minute with 1 mg of CNCbl, 750 nanomoles in the case of AdoCbl and 6750 and 6825 nanomoles per minute in the case of $(CN)_2Cbi$ and $(CN)(H_2O)$ Cbi, respectively [2].

Other features of Cbls include a relatively low cost, nontoxicity, significant thermal resistance capacity due to the large molecular weight and structural complexity and the ability to function in both acidic and alkaline environments.

7.6 Chemistry of the Organometallic Co–C Bond in Vitamin B_{12} Derivatives

AdoCbl and MeCbl are the most biologically active forms of the vitamin B_{12} (CNCbl) family where the cyano group is replaced by 5-deoxyadenosyl and methyl groups, respectively. They act as cofactors (coenzymes) in enzymatic reactions, such as rearrangement and methyl transfer processes occurring in living systems, by intimately binding to the actual enzymes and subsequently interacting with substrate molecules [2, 31, 34–38]. However, the catalytic activity of these vitamin B_{12} coenzymes depends on the behaviour of the organometallic Co–C bond. AdoCbl and MeCbl do not show catalytic activity without the cleavage of this bond. The reversibility of the Co–C bond cleavage allows these coenzymes to undergo a temporary structural and chemical change during the reaction and reassume their original structures when the reaction has completed. AdoCbl undergoes a reversible Co^{3+} to Co^{2+} reduction through homolysis of the Co–C bond, whereas MeCbl undergoes a Co^{3+} to Co^{+} transition type by means of heterolytic cleavage of the bond (Scheme 7.1) [2, 31].

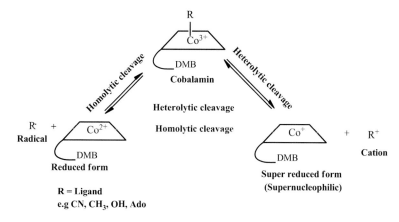

Scheme 7.1 Homolytic and heterolytic Co–C bond cleavages in cobalamins.

Prior to Co–C bond cleavage, the Co atom has a d^6 electronic configuration. However, reduction to the +2 or +1 oxidation state as a result of cleavage gives rise to the paramagnetic d^7 or the diamagnetic d^8 configuration, respectively, with the Ado radical or the methyl cation.

The Co–C bond is regarded as the most stable natural organometallic bond known because of its unprecedented bond strength. For instance, the Co–C bond dissociation energy (BDE) for isolated Ado–Cbl in solution is 31.4 ± 1.5 kcal mol^{-1}, and the observed rate of homolysis is about 10^{-9} s^{-1} at 25°C, which corresponds to a half-life of 22 years [39, 40]. This implies that the Co–C bond cleavage, which is pivotal to the catalytic activity of Cbls, is a slow process. Thus, for any enzyme to make use of a vitamin B_{12} coenzyme, it must be able to significantly activate the organometallic Co–C bond.

7.7 Factors Controlling the Co–C Bond Cleavage

To better understand the catalytic behaviour of Cbls, it is necessary to examine some of the inherent factors which control the cleavage of the Co–C bond, since their catalytic behaviour depends on the kinetics of this bond cleavage. These factors include:

- Positional influence of neighbouring ligands
- Nature of the ligand
- Presence of an enzyme

7.7.1 Positional Influence of Neighbouring Ligands

Depending on their positions relative to the cobalt centre, ligands in Cbl derivatives are classified into two groups, cis and trans ligands for ligands occupying the cis and trans positions, respectively, in a Cbl. These positions can influence both the labilisation and the BDE of the Co–C bond [35]. Cis ligands are fused macrocyclic equatorial ligands which are coordinated to the Co atom through the lone pairs of four nitrogen atoms. They include corrin, corrole, cobaloxime and porphyrin rings (Fig. 7.4). Trans ligands are the ones which are axial or perpendicular to the plane of the corrin unit (Fig. 7.3). A transposition is a position just below the Co centre at a bond angle of about 180° to the beta ligand (Fig. 7.3). In Fig. 7.3, the transposition is occupied by the alpha ligand; hence, trans ligands are also referred

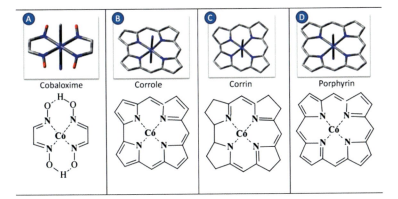

Figure 7.4 Common macrocyclic equatorial ligands [35].

to as trans alpha ligands [35]. On the other hand, the cis positions are occupied by the four equatorial N atoms attached to the Co centre of the corrin ring. The influence of these positions on Co–C bond labilisation and the BDE is discussed in the following sections.

7.7.1.1 Trans influence of the alpha axial ligand

The influence of the trans alpha ligand on Co–C bond cleavage could be electronic and/or steric in nature, depending on the nature and size of the ligand. Increasing the electronic effect by replacing a neutral trans alpha ligand with a charged counterpart of an identical donor atom brings about contraction of the lower axial Co–N bond (i.e. the bond to the alpha ligand in Fig. 7.3B) and elongation of the upper axial Co–C bond (i.e. the bond to the beta ligand in Fig. 7.3B). Elongation of the Co–C bond weakens the bond and, as a result, lowers the BDE. The extent of the lowering depends on the degree of contraction of the lower axial bond. A lower BDE implies that the rupture of the Co–C bond is a rapid process. The lengthening of the Co–C bond and the consequent shortening of the Co–N bond are described as a normal trans influence. An example of this is the Co–C bond-weakening effect of NH_3, NH_2^- and NH^{2-} [35].

On the contrary, the effect of steric hindrance of the alpha axial ligands on Co–C bond weakening is minimal. However, this effect was first considered significant when an increase in the size of the alpha axial ligand was found to produce inverse trans effects between the beta and alpha axial ligands. An inverse trans effect implies that both Co–C and Co–N bonds lengthen and weaken as the bulkiness of the alpha axial ligand increases [35]. However, recent findings on the trans influence of NH_3, NH_2CH_3 and $NH(CH_3)_2$ on the lengths and dissociation energies of both Co–C and Co–N bonds [35] revealed that the elongation of the Co–C bond and the consequent decrease in the BDE as bulkiness increases from NH_3 to $NH(CH_3)_2$ are predominantly due to the trans inductive effect of the ligands rather than their steric effect. This was observed when the Co–N bond was constrained to a fixed bond length to monitor changes in the Co–C bond length only. The corrin ring was populated with more electrons as the number of the methyl groups surrounding the alpha ligand increased. As a result, a trans inductive effect was imposed on the beta ligand (i.e. the upper axial ligand), causing it to shift away from the Co atom, leading to elongation of the Co–C bond. Absence of distortion in the corrin ring serves as additional evidence that confirms no contribution from steric effect [35].

7.7.1.2 Cis influence of the equatorial ligand

The type of macrocycle (ring) coordinated to the Co atom could also impact homolysis of the Co–C bond. Different equatorial ligands alter the Co–C bond length and BDE differently irrespective of the nature of the alpha axial ligand involved. For example, in a study of effects of the equatorial ligands shown in Fig. 7.4, the corrole macrocycle was found to produce the shortest Co–C bond length and, hence, the largest Co–C BDE [35], while both porphyrin and the corrin ring produced the longest Co–C bond and, hence, the least BDE with different alpha axial ligands. Because of its relatively large aromatic ring size, which gives extra stabilisation to the charged ligand, porphyrin gave the least Co–C BDE with NH_2^- as the alpha axial ligand, whereas corrin produced the smallest BDE with NH_3 [35]. In the latter case, the Co centre was drifted closer to the defined mean plane of the corrin unit because of a weak orbital overlap between the metal centre and the beta axial ligand. This resulted in a weaker Co–C bond with a lower BDE.

7.7.2 Nature of the Alpha Axial Ligand

The chemical nature of the alpha ligand in terms of its capacity to donate an electron lone pair into the valence orbital of the cobalt centre also plays a key role in the homolysis of the Co–C bond. Alpha ligands bearing –S, –O and –N as their donor atoms are classified as soft, hard and intermediate ligands, respectively [35]. Soft ligands weaken the Co–C bond, while hard ones strengthen the bond. Intermediate ligands produce a Co–C bond of moderate strength/ stability which is suitable for the catalytic purpose. This explains why nature prefers an intermediate (i.e. N donor atom) ligand in the form of imidazole or histidine as the alpha axial ligand in vitamin B_{12} coenzymes, as opined by Penny (2013) [35].

7.7.3 Presence of an Enzyme

Under normal conditions, homolysis of the Co–C bond is usually the rate-limiting step in Cbl-mediated processes because it is the slowest step [39, 40]. However, the presence of an enzyme could speed up the rate of Co–C bond cleavage to an extent that it is no longer rate-determining [40]. For example, in the study of glutamate mutase-assisted cleavage of the AdoCbl Co–C bond [40], the presence of this enzyme has a dramatic impact on the process. The BDE decreased from 142 kJ/mol in vacuum to 8 kJ/mol in the enzyme (i.e. a reduction of 134 kJ/mol), while the activation energy also dropped from 130 kJ/mol to 25 kJ/mol in the respective media. Therefore, the Co–C bond cleavage step was not the rate-determining step under this condition, because this step occurred faster than the later steps. The observed catalytic effect of the enzyme is the resultant of the following contributing effects.

7.7.3.1 Caging effect

In the caging effect, the enzyme positions the Ado radical relative to the corrin ring at a distance between 3.2 and 4.2 Å from the Co centre (i.e. Co–C distance of 3.2–4.2 Å) without loss of the electrostatic and van der Waals interactions between the Ado moiety and the corrin ring. This lowers the BDE by ~20 kJ/mol [40].

7.7.3.2 Distortion effect

In this case, the Cbl (i.e. the AdoCbl) is distorted by the enzyme through its ribose unit. This distortion, which is more pronounced in the Co^{3+} state of the Cbl, offers the highest catalytic contribution with about 61 kJ/mol reduction in the BDE. The $Co–N_{Im}$ bond (i.e. the bond between the Co ion and the donor nitrogen atom of the alpha imidazole moiety) (Fig. 7.3) has a negligible contribution to the catalytic effect because the lengthening of this bond only destabilises the coenzyme by less than 4 kJ/mol. This ineffective bond elongation is as a result of the enzyme keeping the Ado group away from the Co centre by steric interactions [40].

7.7.3.3 Mutual stabilisation between the Co^{2+} state and the enzyme

The mutual stabilisation effect between the surrounding enzyme and the dissociated form (i.e. the Co^{2+} state) of the coenzyme through electrostatic and van der Waals interactions leads to a total of 53 kJ/mol reduction in the BDE, where the Co^{2+} and the enzyme are stabilised by 42 kJ/mol and 11 kJ/mol, respectively [40].

7.8 Exercises

1. Citing relevant examples, distinguish between homogeneous and heterogeneous catalyses.
2. In sequential order, highlight the stages involved in a heterogeneous catalysed reaction.
3. Mention five examples of Cbl and use the illustrative chemical equation to explain homolytic and heterolytic Co–C bond cleavages with any two biologically active members.
4. Briefly discuss five reasons why vitamin B_{12} is considered as a good catalyst for organic reactions.
5. (a) List three factors controlling the rupture of the Co–C bond in Cbls.

   (b) Provide a suitable justification for why nature prefers N donor ligands compared to O and S donor counterparts in Cbl derivatives.

   (c) Explain the following types of ligand effects as related to Co–C bond cleavage:
   - (i)   inverse trans effect,
   - (ii) trans inductive effect,
   - (iii) caging effect and
   - (iv) distortion effect.

References

1. P. W. van Leeuwen, *Homogeneous Catalysis: Understanding the Art*, Springer Science & Business Media, 2006.
2. M. Giedyk, K. Goliszewska, D. Gryko, Vitamin B_{12} catalysed reactions, *Chem. Soc. Rev.*, **44** (2015) 3391–3404.
3. S. J. Thomson, G. C. Webb, *Heterogeneous Catalysis*, Wiley, 1968.
4. S. M. George, Introduction: heterogeneous catalysis, *Chem. Rev.*, **95** (1995) 475–476.
5. J. M. Thomas, W. J. Thomas, H. Salzberg, Introduction to the principles of heterogeneous catalysis, *J. Electrochem. Soc.*, **114** (1967) 279C–279C.
6. J. M. Thomas, W. J. Thomas, *Principles and Practice of Heterogeneous Catalysis*, 2nd ed., Wiley-VCH Verlag GmbH & Co., Weinheim, Germany, 2014.

7. S. K. Al-Dawery, Photo-catalyst degradation of tartrazine compound in wastewater using TiO_2 and UV light, *J. Eng. Sci. Technol.*, **8** (2013) 683–691.

8. S. Aggarwal, Photo catalytic degradation of methyl orange by using cds semiconductor nanoparticles photo catalyst, *Int. Res. J. Eng. Technol.*, **3** (2016) 451–454.

9. S. Adhikari, D. Sarkar, Metal oxide semiconductors for dye degradation, *Mater. Res. Bull.*, **72** (2015) 220–228.

10. Y. Anjaneyulu, N. S. Chary, D. S. S. Raj, Decolourization of industrial effluents-available methods and emerging technologies–a review, *Rev. Environ. Sci. Biotechnol.*, **4** (2005) 245–273.

11. M. Castellote, N. Bengtsson, Principles of TiO_2 photocatalysis, in *Applications of Titanium Dioxide Photocatalysis to Construction Materials*, Springer, 2011, pp. 5–10.

12. A. Cavicchioli, I. G. Gutz, Effect of scavengers on the photocatalytic digestion of organic matter in water samples assisted by TiO_2 in suspension for the voltammetric determination of heavy metals, *J. Braz. Chem. Soc.*, **13** (2002) 441–448.

13. V. K. Gupta, R. Jain, A. Nayak, S. Agarwal, M. Shrivastava, Removal of the hazardous dye-tartrazine by photodegradation on titanium dioxide surface, *Mater. Sci. Eng. C*, **31** (2011) 1062–1067.

14. M. Kulkarni, P. Thakur, Photocatalytic degradation and mineralization of reactive textile azo dye using semiconductor metal oxide nano particles, *Int. J. Eng. Res. Gen. Sci.*, **2** (2014) 245–254.

15. L. Mahlalela, L. Dlamini, Enhanced photocatalytic activity of titania in the presence of KNO_3 on the photodegradation of dyes, *Surf. Interfaces*, **1** (2016) 21–28.

16. M. Muhler, J. M. Thomas, W. J. Thomas: Principles and Practice of Heterogeneous Catalysis, VCH, Weinheim, 1997, ISBN 3-527-29239-X, Preis: 88, –DM, *Ber. Bunsenges. Phys. Chem.*, **101** (1997) 1560–1560.

17. G. Haller, W. Delgass, Mechanism in heterogeneous catalysis, *ChemInform*, **17** (1986).

18. R. L. Burwell Jr, Mechanism of heterogeneous catalysts, Northwestern *University, Evanston, IL,* Dept. of Chemistry, 1966.

19. J. De Boer, *The Mechanism of Heterogeneous Catalysis*, Elsevier, Amsterdam, 1960.

20. G. Ertl, Mechanisms of heterogeneous catalysis, in *Reactions at Solid Surfaces*, Wiley, 2009, pp. 123–157.

21. J. De Boer, M. Hermans, J. Vleeskens, The chemisorption and physical adsorption of water on silica. I, Proceedings of the Koninklijke Academie van Wetenschappen. Series B, *Phys. Sci.*, **60** (1957) 45–53.

22. N. H. de Leeuw, S. C. Parker, Effect of chemisorption and physisorption of water on the surface structure and stability of alpha-alumina, *J. Am. Ceram. Soc.*, **82** (1999) 3209–3216.

23. F. C. Tompkins, *Chemisorption of Gases on Metals*, Academic Press, New York, 1978.

24. G. Ertl, M. Neumann, K. Streit, Chemisorption of CO on the Pt (111) surface, *Surf. Sci.*, **64** (1977) 393–410.

25. Y. Hisaeda, H. Shimakoshi, M. Tokunaga, S. Kudo, Photochemical dehalogenation of DDT catalyzed by hydrophobic vitamin B_{12}, *Chem. Commun.*, **10** (2004) 1806–1807.

26. D. M. Smith, B. T. Golding, L. Radom, On the mechanism of action of vitamin B_{12}: theoretical studies of the 2-methyleneglutarate mutase catalyzed rearrangement, *J. Am. Chem. Soc.*, **121** (1999) 1037–1044.

27. P. M. Kozlowski, L. Kale, R. Skeel, M. Bh, R. Brunner, A. Gursoy, N. Krawetz, J. Phillips, A. Shinozaki, K. Varadarajan, K. Schulten, Quantum chemical modeling of Co–C bond activation in B_{12} dependent enzymes, *J. Comput. Phys.*, **151** (2002) 283–312.

28. K. L. Brown, J. Li, Activation parameters for the carbon-cobalt bond homolysis of coenzyme B_{12} induced by the B_{12}-dependent ribonucleotide reductase from lactobacillus leichmannii, *J. Am. Chem. Soc.*, **120** (1998) 9466–9474.

29. T. Andruniow, M. Z. Zgierski, P. M. Kozlowski, Density functional theory analysis of stereoelectronic properties of cobalamins, *J. Phys. Chem. B*, **104** (2000) 10921–10927.

30. H. Shimakoshi, Y. Hisaeda, Environmental-friendly catalysts learned from vitamin B_{12}-dependent enzymes, *TCIMAIL*, **138** (2009) 2–11.

31. B. Kräutler, Cobalt: B_{12} enzymes and coenzymes, in *Encyclopedia of Inorganic and Bioinorganic Chemistry*, Wiley, 2006.

32. K. H. Reddy, Coordination compounds in biology: the chemistry of vitamin B_{12} and model compounds, *ChemInform*, **31** (2000).

33. D. G. Brown, The chemistry of vitamin B_{12} and related inorganic model systems, in *Progress in Inorganic Chemistry: Current Research Topics in Bioinorganic Chemistry*, Vol. **18** (1973) pp. 177–286.

34. K. H. Reddy, Coordination compounds in biology, *Resonance*, **4** (1999) 67–77.

35. P. P. Govender, A DFT study of vitamin B_{12} derivatives, WIReDSpace, 2013.

36. K. Gruber, C. Kratky, Coenzyme B_{12} dependent glutamate mutase, *Curr. Opin. Chem. Biol.*, **6** (2002) 598–603.

37. K. L. Brown, Chemistry and enzymology of vitamin B_{12}, *Chem. Rev.*, **105** (2005) 2075–2150.

38. R. Banerjee, *Chemistry and Biochemistry of B_{12}*, John Wiley & Sons, 1999.

39. B. P. Hay, R. G. Finke, Thermolysis of the cobalt-carbon bond of adenosylcobalamin. 2. Products, kinetics, and cobalt-carbon bond dissociation energy in aqueous solution, *J. Am. Chem. Soc.*, **108** (1986) 4820–4829.

40. K. P. Jensen, U. Ryde, How the Co–C bond is cleaved in coenzyme B_{12} enzymes: a theoretical study, *J. Am. Chem. Soc.*, **127** (2005) 9117–9128.

Chapter 8

Vitamin B$_{12}$–Catalysed Reactions

8.1 Introduction

Vitamin B$_{12}$ (cobalamin [Cbl]) serves as a cofactor for Cbl-dependent enzymes such as adenosylcobalamin (AdoCbl) and methylcobalamin (MeCbl) in a range of important biological processes which include nervous system coordination, red blood cell biosynthesis, DNA synthesis and regulation [1]. It plays a vital role in enzymatic processes such as methyl transfer, isomerisation and dehalogenation [2]. The main biologically active forms of the vitamin which act as co-catalysts are AdoCbl and MeCbl [1, 3, 4]. AdoCbl undergoes a reversible homolysis of the Co^{3+}–C bond to form the nucleophilic Co^{2+} state and a 5-deoxyadenosyl (Ado) radical (Scheme 8.1), which is needed for enzymatic isomerisation or rearrangement reactions. MeCbl, on the other hand, undergoes heterolysis of the Co^{3+}–C bond to yield the supernucleophilic Co^+ state and a methyl cation (Scheme 8.2a), which is required for enzymatic methyl transfer reactions. The Co^+ state itself can act as a dehalogenation agent by abstracting an alkyl or halide ion from alkyl halides (Scheme 8.3a,b).

Molecular Modelling of Vitamin B$_{12}$ and Its Analogues
Penny Poomani Govender, Francis Opoku, Olaide Olalekan Wahab, and Ephraim Muriithi Kiarii
Copyright © 2022 Jenny Stanford Publishing Pte. Ltd.
ISBN 978-981-4877-58-9 (Hardcover), 978-1-003-21339-0 (eBook)
www.jennystanford.com

8.2 Vitamin B$_{12}$ Enzymes and Their Functions

Vitamin B$_{12}$ enzymes can be classified into four major groups: B$_{12}$-binding and B$_{12}$-transporting proteins, methyltransferases, corrinoid dehalogenases and Cbl-dependent enzymes [3]. Members of all groups of the vitamin B$_{12}$ enzymes are essential to microorganisms, while B$_{12}$-binding proteins and methyltransferases (such as methylmalonyl-CoA-mutase [MMCM] and methionine synthase) play crucial roles in human and animal metabolism [5, 6].

8.2.1 B$_{12}$-Binding and B$_{12}$-Transporting Proteins

This class of vitamin B$_{12}$ enzymes is essential in human, animal and microorganism metabolic processes, serving as intracellular, membrane-bound and extracellular proteins [3]. The vitamin B$_{12}$-binding protein in humans is a glycoprotein with high binding potential for all Cbls. This protein is secreted in the gastric mucosa. It binds Cbls and transports them to the ileum part of the small intestine, where they are received by receptor proteins for onward transfer across the epithelial absorptive cells in the intestine [3], and then through the blood to specific body cells. Lack of vitamin B$_{12}$-binding extracellular protein causes a disorder in the absorption of Cbl derivatives from nutrition. Hence, it has been widely identified recognised as the cause of pernicious anaemia [3, 7].

8.2.2 Methyltransferases

These are corrinoid enzymes which facilitate methyl transfer processes in human, animal and bacteria metabolism. An example of such a process is Cbl- or cobamide-dependent methylation of homocysteine to methionine [5, 8]. Members of this group of enzymes include methionine synthase, which oversees the synthesis of methionine from methylation of homocysteine; corrinoid enzymes in bacterial acetate metabolism, which act as functional intermediates during autotrophic fixation of CO_2 through acetyl coenzyme A [9, 10]; and the ones in bacterial methanogenesis, which control the formation of methane in methanogenic bacteria [3, 5]. The catalytically active forms of these enzymes are the ones with Co^+-corrins, such as Co^+-Cbl, and methyl-Co^{3+}-corrins, such as MeCbl.

8.2.3 Cobalamin-Dependent Enzymes

Cbl-dependent enzymes are further classified as Cbl-dependent mutases (e.g. glutamate mutase, methylmalonyl-CoA mutase, methylene glutarate mutase, isobutyryl-CoA mutase) [5, 11], deaminases (e.g. ethanol-amine ammonia-lyase and two amino mutases) [3, 5], dehydratases (e.g. diol and glycerol dehydratases), reductive dehalogenases [1] and ribonucleotide reductases [3]. Mutases catalyse isomerisation/rearrangement processes, deaminases control the deamination reaction, dehydratases catalyse the removal of water molecules from diols or glycerol, reductive dehalogenases facilitate the removal of halogen groups (dehalogenation) and ribonucleotide reductases catalyse the reduction of ribonucleotides, which provides building blocks for DNA synthesis.

8.3 Cobalamin-Mediated Organic Reactions

Due to their natural availability, nontoxicity and environmentally friendly nature, Cbls and their synthetic analogues such as cobyrinates have been successfully employed as co-catalysts for the following types of Co-mediated organic reactions:

- Rearrangement
- Methyl transfer
- Dehalogenation
- C–C and C–X multiple bond hydrogenation
- 1,4-addition to the double bond
- Ring-opening reaction
- Cyclopropanation
- Coupling reaction
- Oxidation
- Ring expansion

8.3.1 Rearrangement (Isomerisation)

The AdoCbl-catalysed rearrangement reaction is initiated by homolysis of the Co–C bond to generate the Ado radical and the Co^{2+} state, which can be stabilised by mutual interaction between AdoCbl and the surrounding enzyme. The Ado radical abstracts hydrogen from the substrate to form a substrate radical, which isomerises into a new isomer known as the product radical. The product radical then regenerates the Ado radical through hydrogen abstraction. The final step is the recombination between the Ado radical and the corrin Co^{2+}. The following chemical equations show the steps involved in a typical AdoCbl-catalysed rearrangement process. Notice the change in the positions of X and H between the substrate and the product after rearrangement (Scheme 8.1).

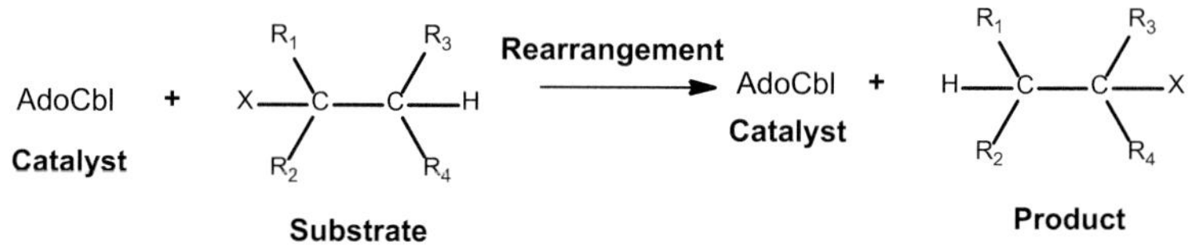

Scheme 8.1 Adenosylcobalamin-catalysed isomerisation/rearrangement reaction.

X is any group other than hydrogen (e.g. –OH, –COOH, halide ions [F^-, Cl^-, Br^- and I^-]), and
R1–R4 could be hydrogen, an alkyl or an acyl group.

Reaction steps:

1. AdoCbl undergoes Co–C bond homolysis.

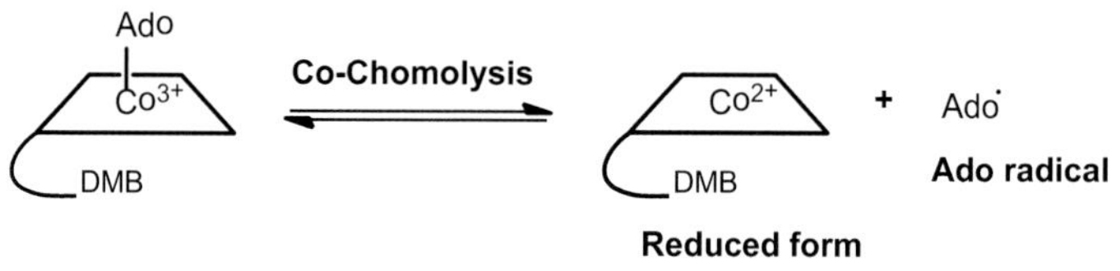

2. The Ado radical abstracts hydrogen from the substrate.

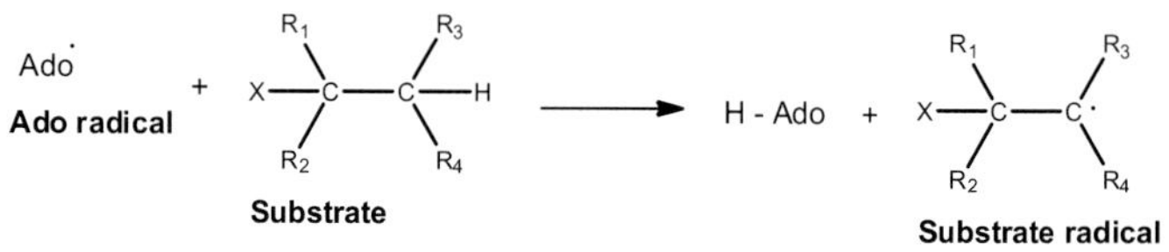

3. The substrate radical isomerises to form a product radical.

Substrate radical → Rearrangement/Isomerisation → **Product radical**

4. The Ado· radical is regenerated by the product radical.

H - Ado + **Product radical** → **Product** + Ado· **Ado radical**

5. AdoCbl is regenerated.

Co^{2+} **DMB** / **Reduced form** + Ado· **Ado radical** → Ado—Co^{3+} **DMB** / **AdoCbl**

8.3.2 Methyl Transfer Reaction (Transmethylation)

The methionine synthase–catalysed transmethylation reaction is facilitated by MeCbl, which serves as a methylating agent for a nucleophilic methyl acceptor. The catalytic cycle consists of the following steps:

1. First, MeCbl undergoes heterolysis of the Co–C bond in the presence of a reducing agent to generate a methyl cation and the Co^+ state.
2. The methyl cation generated is then transferred to a methyl acceptor (a nucleophile), forming a methylated product.
3. Finally, the Co^+ state abstracts a methyl group from a methyl donor, such as methyltetrahydrofolate, to regenerate the coenzyme (i.e. MeCbl).

Example 8.1: MeCbl-catalysed methylation of 2-ammonio-4-mercaptobutanoate

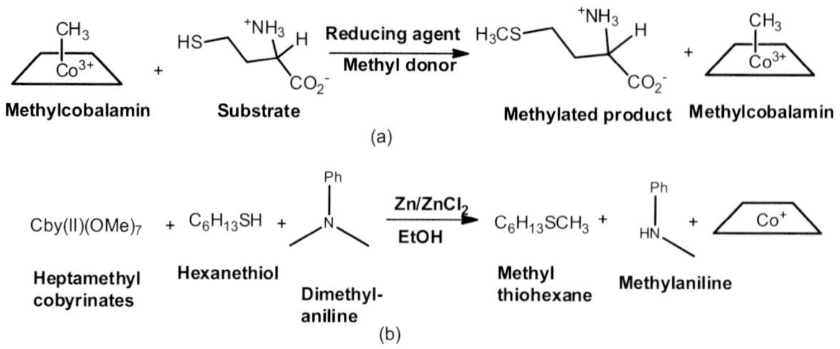

Vitamin B₁₂–Catalysed Reactions

Scheme 8.2 (a) Methylcobalamin-catalysed transmethylation reaction. (b) Heptamethylcobyrinate (Cby(II)OCH₃)₇)-catalysed methyl transfer reaction.

Reaction steps:

1. Heterolysis of the Co–C bond of MeCbl occurs.

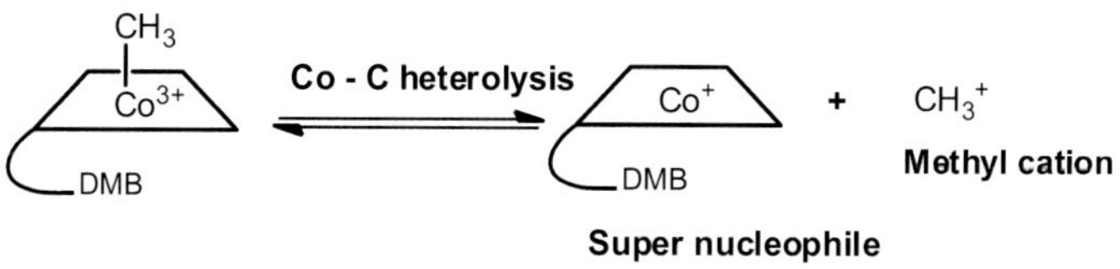

2. There is an electrophilic attack of methyl cation on 2-ammonio-4-mercaptobutanoate, leading to displacement of the hydrogen atom.

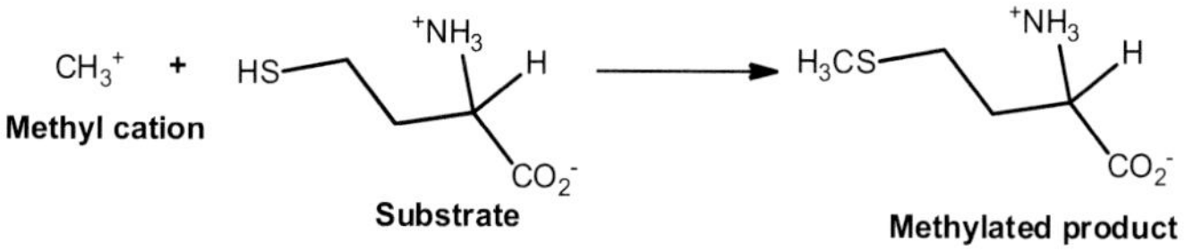

3. The methyl group from a methyl donor is transferred to the supernucleophilic Co⁺.

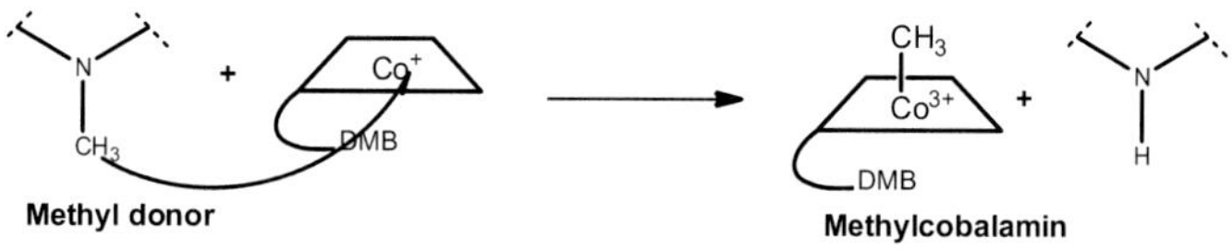

Example 8.2: Heptamethylcobyrinate $(Cby(II)(OMe)_7)$-catalysed methylation of 1-hexanethiol in ethanol by N,N-dimethylaniline in the presence of Zn and $ZnCl_2$. N,N-dimethylaniline is the methyl donor, while Zn and $ZnCl_2$ act as reducing agents.

Reaction steps:

1. Co^{3+} in Cby(II)(OMe)$_7$ is reduced to the Co^+ state.

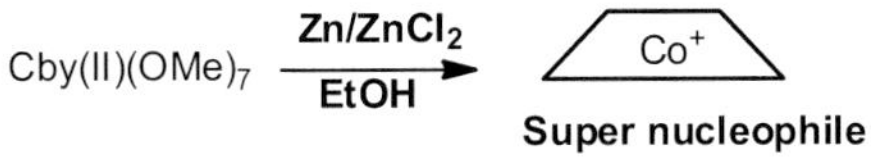

Cby(II)(OMe)$_7$ $\xrightarrow[\text{EtOH}]{\text{Zn/ZnCl}_2}$ [Co^+]

Super nucleophile

2. A methyl group is abstracted from *N,N*-dimethylaniline by Co^+.

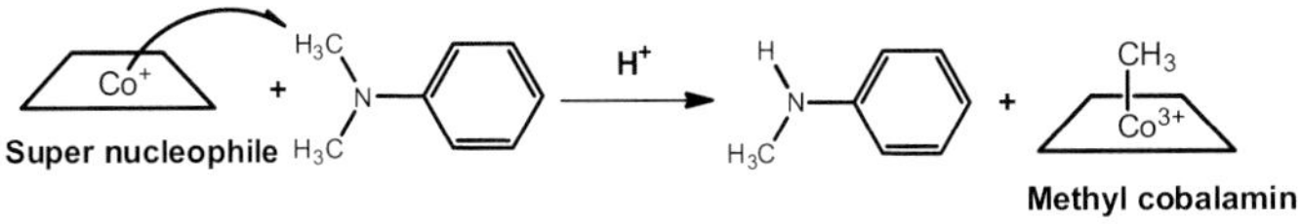

Super nucleophile   **Methyl cobalamin**

3. The hexane thiol is methylated by MeCbl.

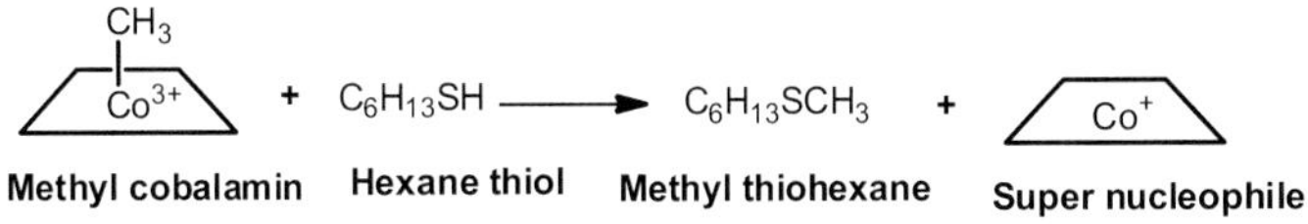

[CH_3 — Co^{3+}] + $C_6H_{13}SH$ ⟶ $C_6H_{13}SCH_3$ + [Co^+]

Methyl cobalamin   **Hexane thiol**   **Methyl thiohexane**   **Super nucleophile**

An important application of the transmethylation reaction is the conversion of arsenic trioxide (As_2O_3) to the less toxic trimethyl arsine oxide using MeCbl [12].

8.3.3   Dehalogenation

Cbl-catalysed removal of halogen substituents from organic halides is one of the most important types of vitamin B_{12}–catalysed reactions which have received immense research attention over the years. This is due to its potential application in the treatment of persistent polyhalogenated environmental pollutants. The widely accepted catalytic cycle begins with the reduction of Co^{3+} to the supernucleophilic Co^+, which subsequently reacts with an electrophilic halide to form an alkylated product (alkylcobalamin) and a free halide ion (Scheme 8.3a). Alternatively, dehalogenation can also occur through halide ion abstraction from the alkyl halide by the supernucleophilic Co^+ to yield an alkyl cation and halocobalamin (i.e. Cbl–X, where X = F⁻, Cl⁻ or Br⁻) (Scheme 8.3b). In other words, the abstracted halide ion does not exist as a free ion but binds to the Cbl moiety [13].

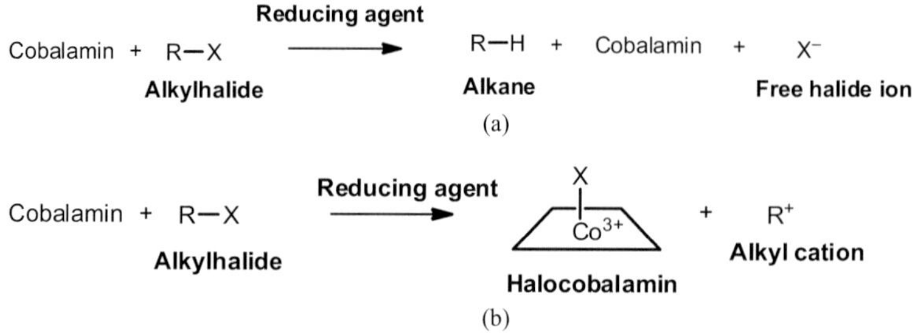

Scheme 8.3

Cobalamin + R—X (Alkylhalide) →[Reducing agent] R—H (Alkane) + Cobalamin + X⁻ (Free halide ion)

(a)

Cobalamin + R—X (Alkylhalide) →[Reducing agent] Halocobalamin (X–Co³⁺) + R⁺ (Alkyl cation)

(b)

Scheme 8.3 Cobalamin-catalysed dehalogenation of alkyl halide to corresponding (a) alkane and free halide ion and (b) halocobalamin and free alkyl cation.

An alternate dehalogenation mechanism is as follows:

1. Co^{3+} in Cbl is reduced to Co^+.

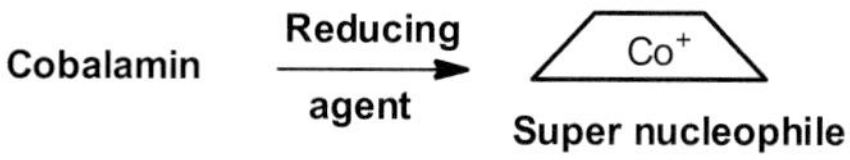

Cobalamin →[Reducing agent] Co^+ (Super nucleophile)

- Co^+ attack an electrophilic halide.

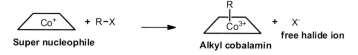

Co^+ (Super nucleophile) + R—X → R–Co^{3+} (Alkyl cobalamin) + X⁻ (free halide ion)

- The Co^{3+}–R bond is homolysed.

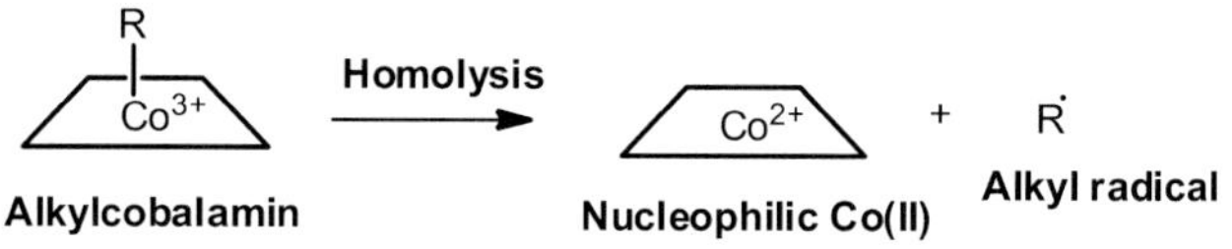

R–Co^{3+} (Alkylcobalamin) →[Homolysis] Co^{2+} (Nucleophilic Co(II)) + Ṙ (Alkyl radical)

- The hydrogen from the solvent is abstracted by a generated alkyl radical.

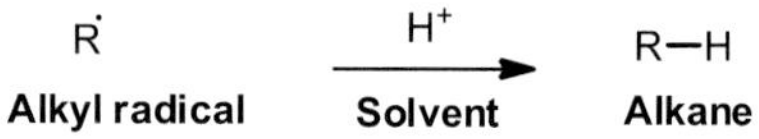

Ṙ (Alkyl radical) →[H⁺ Solvent] R—H (Alkane)

For polyhalogenated compounds, the dehalogenation cycle can be repeated by the nucleophilic Co^{2+} formed as many times as possible to form other dehalogenated products.

A similar mechanism holds for Scheme 8.3b, except that in this case, the supernucleophile is attacked by the halogen group instead of the alkyl group.

Here are a few specific examples of Cbl-catalysed dehalogenation reactions:

- Successive dechlorination of CCl_4 to its trichloro, dichloro and monochloro forms proceeds as follows:

1. The supernucleophilic Co^+ are formed.

Methylcobalamin — Reducing agent — Super nucleophile + CH_3^+ Methyl cation

2. The supernucleophile attacks methyl tetrachloride to yield trichloromethyl Cbl and a free chloride ion.

Super nucleophile + Methyl tetrachloride → Trichloromethyl cobalamin + Cl^- free chloride ion

3. MeCbl is regenerated from trichloromethyl cobalamin. The trichloromethyl radical abstracts a proton from the solvent to give trichloromethane.

Trichloromethyl cobalamin + CH_3^+ Methyl cation — Solvent → Methyl cobalamin + Trichloromethane

These steps are repeated with trichloromethane to furnish the dichloro product, which also follows the same steps to yield the monochloro product.

- Stereoselective dechlorination of tetrachloroethylene to Z-1,2-dichloroethylene in the presence of titanium(III) citrate as a reducing agent [14–16]

Tetrachloroethylene — Cobalamin / Ti(III) citrate → Trichloroethylene — Cobalamin / Ti(III) citrate → Dichloroethylene

- Defluorination of 2,3,3,3-tetrafluoropropene using titanium(III) citrate as a reducing agent in the presence of cyanocobalamin (CNCbl) [17]

Tetrafluoropropene → Trifluoropropene → Difluoropropene

(CNCbl / Ti(III) citrate)

An important application of Cbl-catalysed dehalogenation is the dechlorination of lindane using aquacobalamin (H_2OCbl), MeCbl or aquacyanocobalamin [(CN)(H_2O)Cbl] in the presence of reducing agents such as titanium(III) citrate, dithiothreitol and cysteine [12, 18].

For Cbl-catalysed dehalogenation reactions involving solvents of low polarity, such as tetrahydrofuran (THF), acetone, toluene, dichloromethane (DCM), etc., where most of the Cbls are less soluble, hydrophobic cobyrinates, such as heptamethylcobyrinate [Cby(II) $(OMe)_7$] and dicyanoheptamethylcobyrinate [$(CN)_2$Cby$(OMe)_7$], can be employed instead of the actual Cbls [19]. Cobyrinates are derivatives of Cbls which contain peripheral ester groups around the corrin macrocycle [1].

8.3.4 C–C and C–X Multiple Bond Hydrogenation

Hydrogenation refers to the addition of hydrogen molecules across multiple bonds of an unsaturated substrate. A reducing agent supplies the needed hydrogen molecules, which bring about an increase in the saturation of the substrate. Hydrogenation processes can be catalysed by the addition of some Cbl derivatives such as H_2OCbl and CNCbl. In the presence of a reducing agent and sufficient amount of Cbl in a protic solvent, activated olefins, such as α,β-unsaturated carbonyl compounds, nitriles, nitro compounds, etc., can add hydrogen molecules across their carbon–carbon multiple bond and/or their carbon–heteroatom bond [20, 21]. Examples of such reactions include H_2OCbl-catalysed reduction of nitriles to corresponding aldehydes [22] and CNCbl-catalysed hydrogenation of prochiral alkenes [21]. Prochiral molecules are achiral molecules which can be converted to their chiral forms in a single step through the formation of a new stereogenic carbon during a reaction [23].

- H_2OCbl-catalysed nitrile reduction

Cobalamin-Mediated Organic Reactions | 101

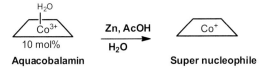

(a)

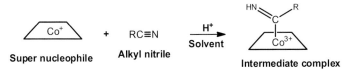

(Z)-ethyl-3-methyl-5-phenylpent-2-enoate   (S)-ethyl-3-methyl-5-phenylpentanoate
(A prochiral substrate)

(b)

Scheme 8.4 (a) Aquacobalamin-catalysed reduction of nitrile to the corresponding aldehyde.

Only aliphatic nitriles undergo this reaction. No evidence of reduction was observed for the aromatics [22]. (b) Cyanocobalamin-catalysed hydrogenation of (Z)-ethyl-3-methyl-5-phenylpent-2-enoate to (S)-ethyl-3-methyl-5-phenylpentanoate.

Reaction steps:

1. A supernucleophile is formed from H_2OCbl.

2. The supernucleophile attacks the nitrile, accompanied by proton abstraction from the solvent to form an intermediate complex.

Note: Observe the occurrence of the first hydrogen atom addition in the intermediate complex.

3. The intermediate complex is reduced, followed by hydrolysis to produce an aldehyde.

102 | Vitamin B_{12}–Catalysed Reactions

Note: Observe the second hydrogen atom addition in the reduced nitrile.

- CNCbl-catalysed hydrogenation of prochiral alkenes: In this reaction, a supernucleophilic Cbl(I) ion is first formed through a reductive cleavage of the Co–C bond of CNCbl. This supernucleophile preferentially attacks the *re* side of the prochiral substrate, forming a new Co–C bond with the substrate. This is then followed by reductive cleavage of the new Co–C bond formed with retention of the initial configuration.

Reaction steps:

1. A supernucleophile is formed from CNCbl.

2. The supernucleophile attacks from the *re* side of the substrate to form an intermediate complex.

3. The intermediate complex is reduced to the product.

Note: Reduction in the above cases is in terms of addition of hydrogen.

8.3.5 1,4-Addition to Double Bonds

Vitamin B_{12}-mediated double-bond hydrogenation usually takes place in a protic solvent (Section 8.2.4). However, when an aprotic environment is introduced together with an alkyl halide which acts as a potential source of radical, a 1,4-addition to the double bond is observed (Scheme 8.5a–c). Examples of this type of reaction are as follows:

- H_2OCbl-catalysed cyclisation of bromoalkylcyclohexenone in the presence of 6-bromoalkyne as a potential radical source [19]: This is a type of intramolecular 1,4-addition reaction which produces bicyclic products under a chemical or electrochemical condition. The cyclisation can yield six- and seven-membered rings through an endocyclic closure mechanism in which the component rings of the resulting bicyclic compound are fused together, or five- and six-membered rings through an exocyclic closure mechanism in which the component rings are connected by one carbon atom (Scheme 8.5b).

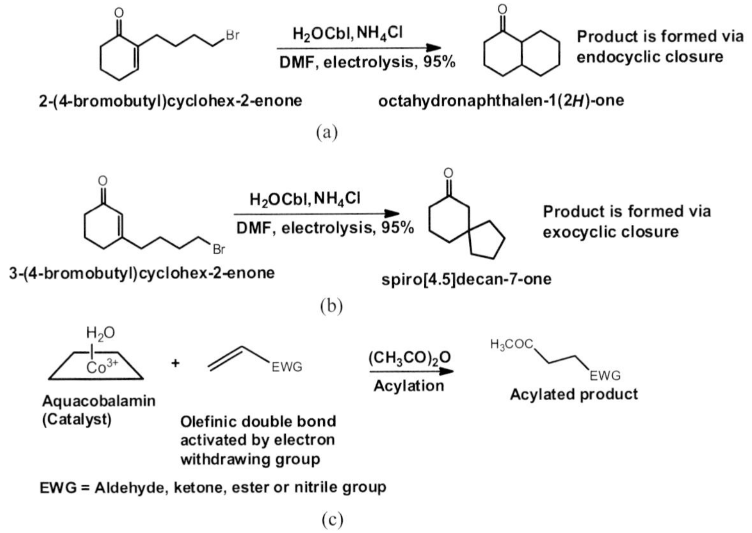

Scheme 8.5 Aquacobalamin-catalysed intramolecular 1,4-addition reaction (a) of 2-(4-bromobutyl)cyclohexenone to octahydronaphthalenone, (b) of 3-(4-bromobutyl)cyclohexenone to spirodecan-7-one and (c) between carboxylic anhydride α,β–unsaturated aldehydes, ketones, nitriles or esters.

Absence of evidence for the formation of tertiary alcohols through a hydrogen attack on the carbonyl group of the reactant confirms the non-occurrence of hydrogenation due to the use of an aprotic solvent.

- H$_2$OCbl-catalysed intermolecular 1,4-addition of carboxylic anhydride to α,β-unsaturated aldehydes, ketones, nitriles or esters [19]: This reaction involves the formation of acetylcobalamin through the attack of an acetyl radical generated from the anhydride on supernucleophilic Cbl(I). The acetylcobalamin releases the acetyl radical on photolysis, which causes acylation of the activated olefinic double bond [24] (Scheme 8.5c).

Reaction steps:

1. The Co–C bond is heterolytically cleaved to form the super-reduced Cbl(I) state.

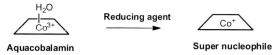

Aquacobalamin   Super nucleophile

2. An acetyl radical is generated, with a subsequent attack of the radical on the supernucleophile.

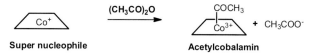

Super nucleophile   Acetylcobalamin

3. The activated olefin substrate is acylated.

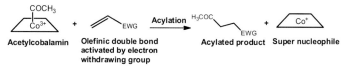

Acetylcobalamin   Olefinic double bond   Acylated product Super nucleophile
                  activated by electron
                  withdrawing group

EWG = Aldehyde, ketone, ester or nitrile group

The electron-withdrawing group (EWG) could be an aldehyde, a ketone, a nitrile or an ester functional group.

8.3.5.1 Scheffold principles of cobalamin-mediated 1,4-addition reactions [25]

For any cobalt complex catalyst to be considered suitable for C–C bond formation reactions under reducing conditions, the following criteria must be met:

- It should be able to switch easily between its Co(III) form and its corresponding super-reduced Co(I) state.
- The Co(I) complexes should exhibit high nucleophilicity at the Co centre and readily form organometallic intermediates which contain a Co–C bond with alkyl, vinyl and acyl derivatives in rapid reactions.
- The Co–C bond of the organometallic intermediates should be cleaved in a fast reaction with the formation of an active carbon species and a cobalt complex, which has to be recycled to the active Co(I) complex under the same reaction conditions.
- The cobalt complex should exhibit appropriate solubility and stability under the reaction conditions.

8.3.6 Ring-Opening Reactions

Cyclic compounds such as oxiranes, cyclopropanes and aziridines possess a large ring strain and are as a result less stable. They consequently undergo a spontaneous ring-opening reaction in the presence of strong nucleophiles to produce their acyclic analogues. Due to high nucleophilicity of the super-reduced form of vitamin B_{12}, ring-opening reactions of these compounds can be effectively promoted by Cbls. For example, cyclopropanes containing EWGs undergo a spontaneous ring-opening reaction with the supernucleophilic form of CNCbl (Scheme 8.6) [26]. The unsubstituted position in the cyclopropanes is attacked by the supernucleophilic Co^+, forming an alkyl–cobalt(III) complex with cleavage of a C–C bond in the substrate. The alkyl–cobalt complex then undergoes a hydrogen–cobalt elimination reaction to produce the corresponding olefin.

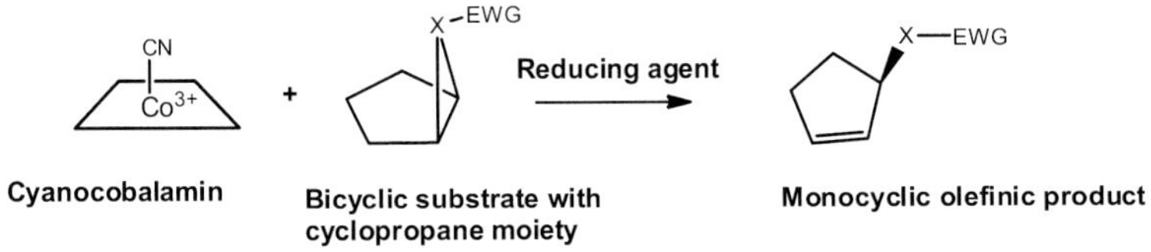

Cyanocobalamin   Bicyclic substrate with cyclopropane moiety   Monocyclic olefinic product

Scheme 8.6 Cyanocobalamin-catalysed ring-opening reaction of the bicyclic substrate containing cyclopropane (X = C) part to the monocyclic olefinic derivative.

Reaction steps:

1. A supernucleophile is formed from CNCbl through heterolytic cleavage of the Co–C bond.

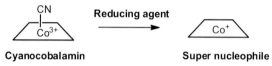

2. The supernucleophile attacks the bicyclic substrate through a cyclopropane (X = C) moiety to form an alkyl–cobalt(III) complex.

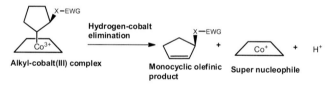

3. The supernucleophile and hydrogen are eliminated to produce an olefinic product.

X = C, O or N for cyclopropane, epoxide or aziridine, respectively.

Cbl-catalysed ring-opening reactions of epoxides (X = O) and aziridines (X = N) proceed via the same mechanism, but the nucleophilic attack of Co⁺ occurs faster on the epoxide ring compared to the aziridine. The hydrogen–cobalt elimination reaction of their respective alkyl–cobalt(III) complexes gives allylic alcohols and amines, respectively, in a nonstereospecific manner.

8.3.7 Coupling Reactions

Both halide coupling and alkene coupling reactions can be catalysed by vitamin B_{12}. The catalytic cycle begins with the formation of alkyl–Cbl derivatives, followed by homolytic cleavage of the Co–C bond to release the alkyl radical, which dimerises into a coupled product.

8.3.7.1 Halide coupling reaction of alkyl halides (Scheme 8.7a)

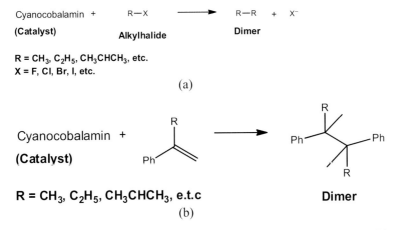

R = CH$_3$, C$_2$H$_5$, CH$_3$CHCH$_3$, e.t.c

Scheme 8.7 (a) Cobalamin-catalysed coupling reaction of alkyl halides and (b) cyanocobalamin-catalysed dimerization of styrene.

Reaction steps:

1. Alkylcobalamin is formed by displacement of a halide ion from the alkyl halide.

   R—X + Co⁺ ⟶ [R–Co³⁺] + X⁻
   Alkylhalide   Super nucleophile   Alkylcobalamin

2. An alkyl radical is generated through homolytic cleavage of the alkylcobalamin Co–C bond.

   [R–Co³⁺] —Co—C Homolysis→ Co²⁺ + Ṙ
   Alkylcobalamin   Nucleophilic Cbl (II)   Alkyl radical

3. The alkyl radical generated is dimerised.

   Ṙ + Ṙ —Dimerisation→ R–R
                          Dimer

8.3.7.2 Alkene coupling reaction of styrene derivatives (Scheme 8.7b)

Reaction steps:

1. An alkylarylcobalamin complex is formed through the attack of supernucleophilic Cbl on the styrene derivative.

Styrene derivative   **Super nucleophile**   **Alkylarylcobalamin**

2. An alkylaryl radical is generated through homolytic cleavage of the alkylarylcobalamin Co–C bond.

Alkylarylcobalamin   **Nucleophilic Cbl (II)**   **Alkylaryl radical**

3. The alkylaryl radical generated is dimerised.

Alkylaryl radical   **Dimer**

The choice of a catalyst and reducing conditions are vital in coupling reactions. The reaction condition must be able to allow spontaneous switching of the vitamin between the Co^{3+} and Co^+ states and also guarantee significant stability of the generated alkyl radical.

For example, CNCbl proved effective for dimerization of benzyl bromide and styrene derivatives in the presence of Ti(III) citrate in aqueous ethanol [1, 14]. The catalyst dosage required for the reactions is relatively high (~10 mol%), and the product yield decreases with benzyl bromide but increases with styrene as R changes from H to CH_3 [1, 14].

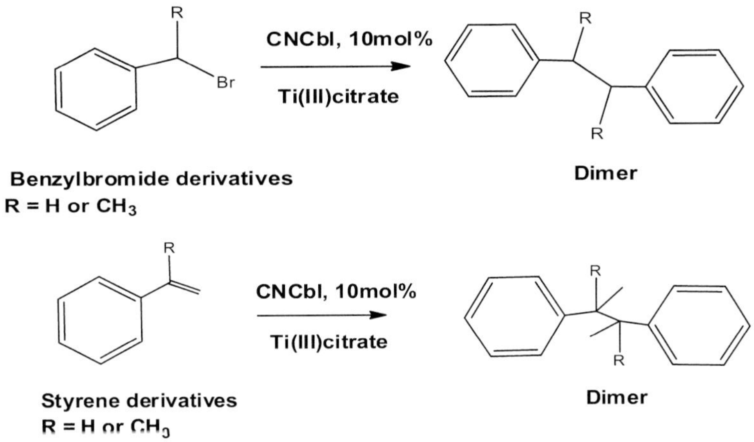

Cobalamin-Mediated Organic Reactions | 109

Benzylbromide derivatives
R = H or CH$_3$

Dimer

Styrene derivatives
R = H or CH$_3$

Dimer

8.3.8 Cyclopropanation

Using CNCbl as a catalyst, tetrachloroalkanols undergoes reductive cyclisation followed by complete dechlorination in the presence of sodium borohydride to produce cyclopropyl-substituted alkanols (Scheme 8.8a), which is a nontoxic derivative [1, 2].

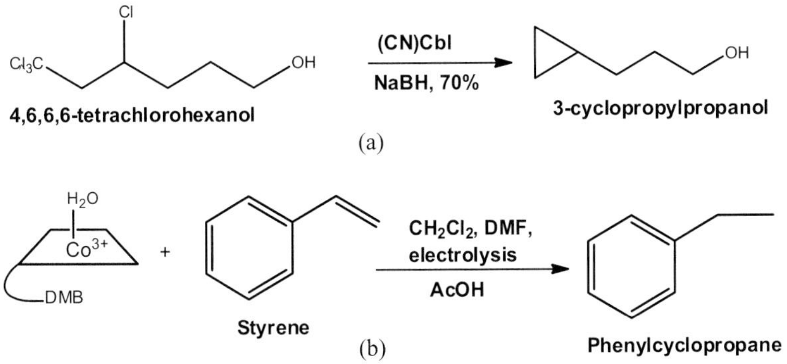

4,6,6-tetrachlorohexanol

3-cyclopropylpropanol

(a)

Styrene

Phenylcyclopropane

(b)

Scheme 8.8 (a) Cyanocobalamin-catalysed cyclisation of tetrachlorohexanol with sodium borohydride to produce cyclopropylpropanol and (b) aquacobalamin-catalysed cyclopropanation of styrene to phenylcyclopropane.

Similarly, H$_2$OCbl-catalysed cyclopropanation of styrene with dichloromethane in dimethylformamide (DMF) predominantly gives a cyclopropane derivative (Scheme 8.8b). The catalytic cycle begins with the production of a Cbl(I) ion by means of electrochemical

Vitamin B_{12}-Catalysed Reactions

induction. The Cbl(I) ion combines with a chloromethylene cation from methylene dichloride, which is then released as a radical through homolytic cleavage of the Co–C bond between Cbl and the attached chloromethylene cation. The resulting chloromethylene radical reacts with the styrene to produce a carbanion, which cyclises into a cyclopropyl-substituted derivative. The carbanion can also be protonated in the solvent medium, but this gives an infinitesimally low yield [1].

Reaction steps:

1. A supernucleophilic Cbl(I) is produced from H_2OCbl.

Aquacobalamin → **Super nucleophile**

2. The chloromethylene cation attacks the supernucleophile to form a chloromethyl–Cbl complex.

Super nucleophile + **Methylene dichloride** → **Chloromethyl cobalamin complex** + **Chlorine radical**

3. The chloromethyl–Cbl complex undergoes Co–C homolysis to produce a chloromethyl radical.

Chloromethylcobalamin complex → **Chloromethyl radical** + **Nucleophilic Cbl**

4. The chloromethyl radical reacts with styrene to form a chlorophenylpropyl radical.

Chloromethyl radical + **Styrene** → **1-chloro-3-phenylpropyl radical**

5. The chlorophenylpropyl radical is reduced to a carbanion, and the carbanion is subsequently cyclised to a cyclopropane derivative.

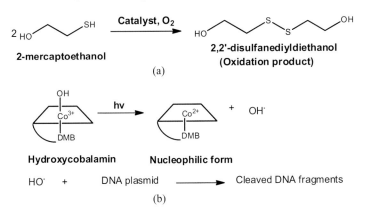

8.3.9 Oxidation

Although the larger percentage of Cbl-catalysed reactions follow the reductive mechanism, where the catalytically active form of the Cbl is the super-reduced Co$^+$ state, there are significant cases of vitamin B$_{12}$-catalysed oxidation reactions in which the Cbl remains in the Co^{3+} state, as follows:

- Vitamin B$_{12}$-catalysed aerobic oxidation of thiols, such as 2-mercaptoethanol (Scheme 8.9a) [27]

Scheme 8.9 (a) Cobalamin- or cobinamide-catalysed oxidation of 2-mercaptoethanol and (b) hydroxycobalamin-mediated DNA plasmid fragmentation.

With either a Cbl or cobinamide series of vitamin B$_{12}$ as a catalyst, the mechanism of the reaction is the same. However, the cobinamide series demonstrated higher catalytic activity compared to the corresponding Cbl series, and the highest catalytic activity was observed in diaquacobinamide $((H_2O)_2Cbi)$ [27]. The catalytic cycle begins with substitution of the beta aqua ligand with a thiol molecule to furnish a Co(III)–S complex. The Co^{3+} in the complex is then reduced to the Co^+ state by the attack of a thiolate anion on the complex, which also leads to the production of a disulphide bond. The catalyst is regenerated in the final step by molecular oxygen.

Reaction steps:

1. A beta aqua ligand is substituted with a thiol molecule.

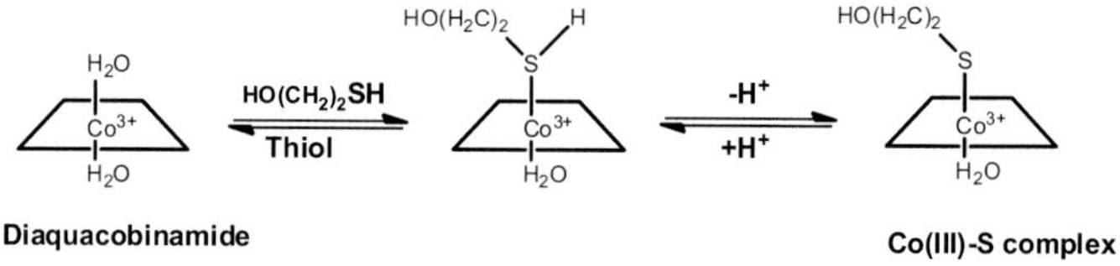

Diaquacobinamide · Co(III)-S complex

2. The Co^{3+} is reduced to Co^+ by the attack of a thiolate ion on the Co(III)–S complex.

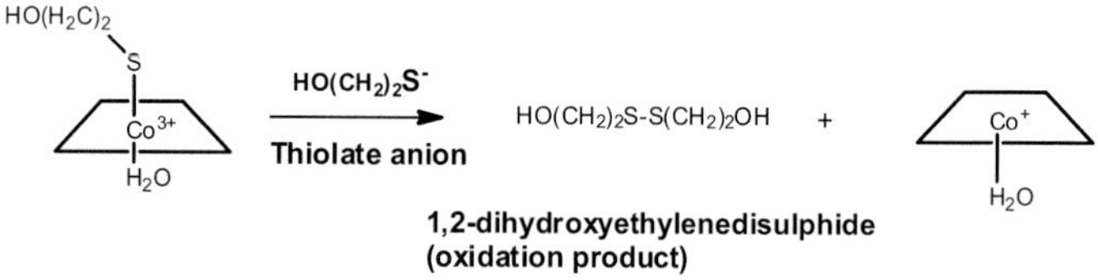

1,2-dihydroxyethylenedisulphide (oxidation product)

3. Diaquacobinamide is regenerated.

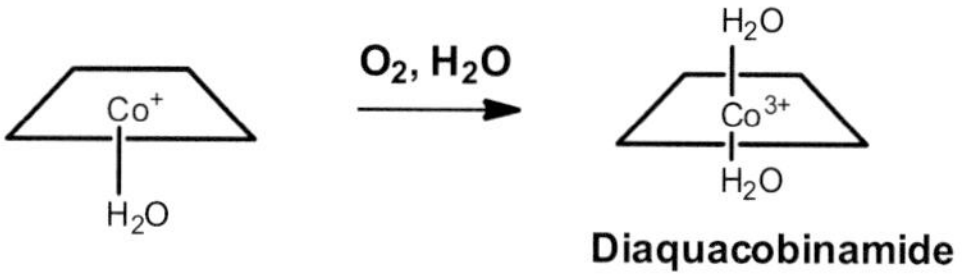

Diaquacobinamide

For catalysts containing beta alkyl ligands, a preliminary step involving light-activated conversion of the Co-alkyl species to the active Co-aqua species is involved [1].

- Hydroxocobalamin (HOCbl)-catalysed hydroxyl radical cleavage of DNA plasmid strands in the presence of light (Scheme 8.9b) [28]

In the presence of the light of sufficient energy, the Co(III)–OH bond in HOCbl undergoes homolysis to release a hydroxyl radical, which subsequently splits the DNA plasmid. The presence of molecular oxygen allows the regeneration of the catalyst.

Cbl-mediated oxidation of organic and inorganic compounds such as hydrazine, nitric oxide and nitrite has also been reported [27, 29].

8.3.10 Ring Expansion Reactions

Ring expansion reactions are an important class of organic reactions used for the synthesis of cyclic compounds, especially when other synthetic routes are difficult for the compound(s) of interest. Tributylstannane (Bu_3SnH) is a known radical promoter for ring expansion reactions. However, the use of this reagent is significantly limited in organic synthesis because it stimulates numerous unwanted side reactions which interfere with ring expansion processes. In contrast, Cbl derivatives serve as a milder and a more eco-friendly alternative. For example, transformation of 2-methyl-1,3-cyclopentanedione to its respective 6-membered cyclic product was achieved in the presence of $Cby(II)(OC_3H_7)_7$ [30] (Scheme 8.10). In this reaction, vanadium trichloride served as a reductant, which enabled the formation of an alkyl–Co(III) complex, and UV radiation assisted Co–C homolysis.

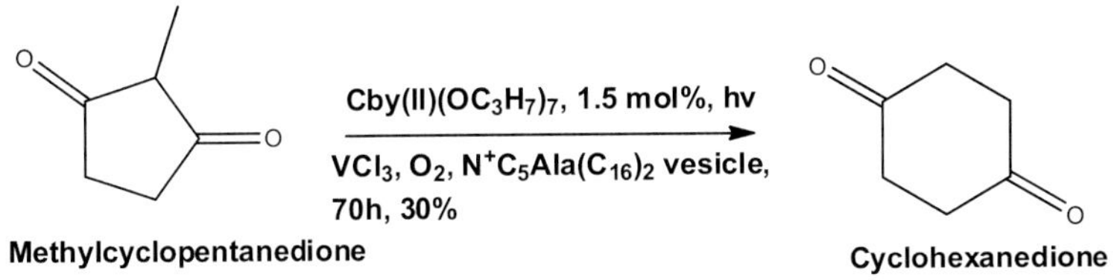

Cby(II)(OC$_3$H$_7$)$_7$, 1.5 mol%, hv

VCl$_3$, O$_2$, N$^+$C$_5$Ala(C$_{16}$)$_2$ vesicle, 70h, 30%

Methylcyclopentanedione

Cyclohexanedione

Scheme 8.10 Heptapropylcobirinate-catalysed ring expansion reaction of methylcyclopentanedione to cyclohexanedione.

8.4 Exercises

1. State four classifications of vitamin B_{12} enzymes and their functions.
2. Highlight six types of organic reactions which can be catalysed by Cbl and its analogues.
3. Explain the following:
   - Cobirinates

114 | *Vitamin B_{12}–Catalysed Reactions*

- Prochiral substrates
- Endocyclic and exocyclic types of ring closure

4. Highlight the steps involved in the following Cbl-catalysed reactions:
   - Isomerisation
   - Transmethylation
   - Dehalogenation
   - Coupling
   - Ring-opening reaction

5. State the conditions necessary for a cobalt complex to be considered suitable for 1,4-addition reactions.

6. Identify the following types of enzyme-catalysed organic reactions and suggest a suitable enzyme for each.

References

1. M. Giedyk, K. Goliszewska, D. Gryko, Vitamin B_{12} catalysed reactions, *Chem. Soc. Rev.*, **44** (2015) 3391–3404.

2. K. L. Brown, Chemistry and enzymology of vitamin B_{12}, *Chem. Rev.*, **105** (2005) 2075–2150.

3. B. Kräutler, Cobalt: B_{12} enzymes and coenzymes, in *Encyclopedia of Inorganic and Bioinorganic Chemistry*, Wiley, 2006.

4. P. P. Govender, A DFT study of vitamin B_{12} derivatives, WIReDSpace, 2013.

5. R. Banerjee, *Chemistry and Biochemistry of B_{12}*, John Wiley & Sons, 1999.

6. B. Kräutler, S. Ostermann, in *The Porphyrin Handbook*, Academic Press, San Diego, 2003.

7. L. J. Machlin, *Handbook of Vitamins: Nutritional, Biochemical, and Clinical Aspects*, Marcel Dekker, 1984.

8. R. G. Matthews, Cobalamin-dependent methyltransferases, *Acc. Chem. Res.*, **34** (2001) 681–689.

9. S. W. Ragsdale, Enzymology of the acetyl-CoA pathway of CO_2 fixation, *Crit. Rev. Biochem. Mol. Biol.*, **26** (1991) 261–300.

10. S. W. Ragsdale, M. Kumar, Nickel-containing carbon monoxide dehydrogenase/acetyl-CoA synthase, *Chem. Rev.*, **96** (1996) 2515–2540.

11. K. Gruber, C. Kratky, Coenzyme B_{12} dependent glutamate mutase, *Curr. Opin. Chem. Biol.*, **6** (2002) 598–603.

12. Y. Hisaeda, H. Shimakoshi, K. Kadish, K. Smith, R. Guilard, *Handbook of Porphyrin Science*, World Scientific Publishing, 2010.

13. K. A. Payne, C. P. Quezada, K. Fisher, M. S. Dunstan, F. A. Collins, H. Sjuts, C. Levy, S. Hay, S. E. Rigby, D. Leys, Reductive dehalogenase structure suggests a mechanism for B_{12}-dependent dehalogenation, *Nature*, **517** (2015) 513.

14. J. Shey, C. M. McGinley, K. M. McCauley, A. S. Dearth, B. T. Young, W. A. Van der Donk, Mechanistic investigation of a novel vitamin B_{12}-catalyzed carbon-carbon bond forming reaction, the reductive dimerization of arylalkenes, *J. Org. Chem.*, **67** (2002) 837–846.

15. D. A. Pratt, W. A. Van Der Donk, On the role of alkylcobalamins in the vitamin B_{12}-catalyzed reductive dehalogenation of perchloroethylene and trichloroethylene, *Chem. Commun.*, (2006) 558–560.

16. S. Kliegman, K. McNeill, Dechlorination of chloroethylenes by cob (I) alamin and cobalamin model complexes, *Dalton Trans.*, (2008) 4191–4201.

17. J. Im, G. E. Walshe-Langford, J.-W. Moon, F. E. Löffler, Environmental fate of the next generation refrigerant 2, 3, 3, 3-tetrafluoropropene (HFO-1234yf), *Environ. Sci. Technol.*, **48** (2014) 13181–13187.

18. T. Marks, J. Allpress, A. Maule, Dehalogenation of lindane by a variety of porphyrins and corrins, *Appl. Environ. Microbiol.*, **55** (1989) 1258–1261.

19. R. Scheffold, S. Abrecht, R. Orlinski, H.-R. Ruf, P. Stamouli, O. Tinembart, L. Walder, C. Weymuth, Vitamin B_{12}-mediated electrochemical reactions in the synthesis of natural products, *Pure Appl. Chem.*, **59** (1987) 363–372.

20. H. Shimakoshi, Y. Hisaeda, B_{12}-TiO_2 hybrid catalyst for light-driven hydrogen production and hydrogenation of C–C multiple bonds, *ChemPlusChem*, **79** (2014) 1250–1253.

21. A. Fischli, J. J. Daly, Cob (I) alamin as catalyst. 8th communication. Cob (I) alamin and heptamethyl cob (I) yrinate during the reduction of α, β-unsaturated carbonyl derivatives, *Helv. Chim. Acta*, **63** (1980) 1628–1643.

22. M. Giedyk, S. Fedosov, D. Gryko, An amphiphilic, catalytically active, vitamin B_{12} derivative, *Chem. Commun.*, **50** (2014) 4674–4676.

23. M. John, *Fundamentals of Organic Chemistry*, Thomson-Brooks/Cole, 2003.

24. L. Walder, R. Orlinski, Mechanism of the light-assisted nucleophilic acylation of activated olefins catalyzed by vitamin B_{12}, *Organometallics*, **6** (1987) 1606–1613.

25. R. Scheffold, G. Rytz, L. Walder, R. Orlinski, Z. Chilmonczyk, Formation of (CC) bonds catalyzed by vitamin B_{12}, *Pure Appl. Chem.*, **55** (1983) 1791–1797.

26. Y. Hisaeda, T. Nishioka, Y. Inoue, K. Asada, T. Hayashi, Electrochemical reactions mediated by vitamin B_{12} derivatives in organic solvents, *Coord. Chem. Rev.*, **198** (2000) 21–37.

27. D. W. Jacobsen, L. S. Troxell, K. L. Brown, Catalysis of thiol oxidation by cobalamins and cobinamides: reaction products and kinetics, *Biochemistry*, **23** (1984) 2017–2025.

28. T. A. Shell, D. S. Lawrence, A new trick (hydroxyl radical generation) for an old vitamin (B12), *J. Am. Chem. Soc.*, **133** (2011) 2148–2150.

29. D. Mimica, F. Bedioui, J. H. Zagal, Reversibility of the L-cysteine/L-cystine redox process at physiological pH on graphite electrodes modified with coenzyme B_{12} and vitamin B_{12}, *Electrochim. Acta*, **48** (2002) 323–329.

30. Y. Murakami, Y. Hisaeda, T. Ohno, Y. Matsuda, Ring-expansion reactions catalyzed by hydrophobic vitamin B_{12} in synthetic bilayer membrane, *Chem. Lett.*, **17** (1988) 621–624.

Chapter 9

Vitamin B$_{12}$ Derivatives

Vitamin B$_{12}$ is a vital nutrient for the body, which is required to support immune function, contribute to red blood cell formation, stimulate serotonin production, protect brain and nerve cells, support energy and protect RNA and DNA. Among all the vitamins, vitamin B$_{12}$ is the most chemically complex. The levels of vitamin B$_{12}$ decrease in our blood as time goes by; therefore, older people are advised to take a supplement to maintain their general well-being. Vitamin B$_{12}$, together with folic acid, helps maintain the heart, as well as aid the process levels of amino acids. Cobalamin is the chemical name of vitamin B$_{12}$ since it is derived from the central cobalt (Co) atom. However, cobalamin cannot be found in its chemically pure form, because it is commonly bound to other molecules. Vitamin B$_{12}$, as a cofactor for methylcobalamin (MeCbl)- and adenosylcobalamin (AdoCbl)-dependent enzymes, play an important role in biological processes, such as DNA regulation and synthesis, red blood cell formation and nervous system function. Biologically active forms of vitamin B$_{12}$, including cyanocobalamin (CNCbl), AdoCbl, hydroxocobalamin (HOCbl) and MeCbl, are complex organometallic molecules because of their distinctive σ Co–C bonds (see Fig. 9.1 and Table 9.1).

Molecular Modelling of Vitamin B$_{12}$ and Its Analogues
Penny Poomani Govender, Francis Opoku, Olaide Olalekan Wahab, and Ephraim Muriithi Kiarii
Copyright © 2022 Jenny Stanford Publishing Pte. Ltd.
ISBN 978-981-4877-58-9 (Hardcover), 978-1-003-21339-0 (eBook)
www.jennystanford.com

Table 9.1   Comparison of the various types of vitamin B$_{12}$

Cobalamin	Natural form	Bioactive coenzyme	Conversion steps necessary	Sustained release	Special effect
Cyanocobalamin	No	No	4	Average to poor	No particular effect
Hydroxocobalamin	Yes	No	3	Good	Detoxification of cyanide and NO
Methylcobalamin	Yes	Yes	0	Average	DNA, brain, nerves, blood, detoxification
Adenosylcobalamin	Yes	Yes	0	Average	Energy, muscles, brain, DNA

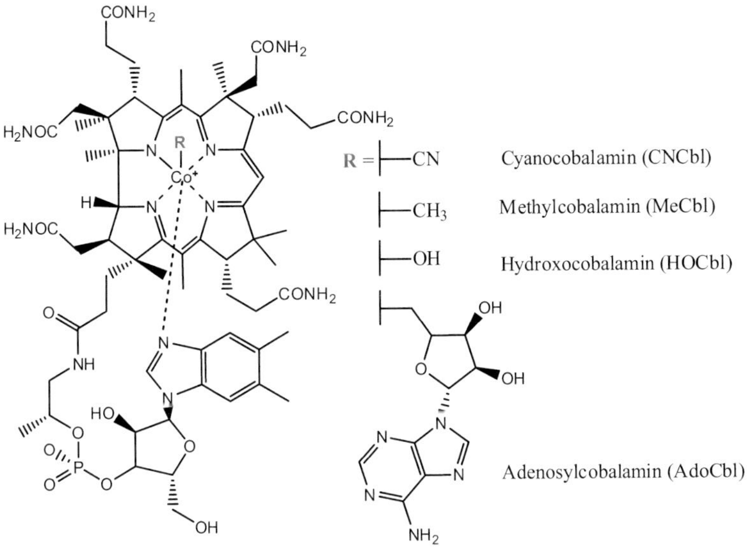

Figure 9.1 Chemical structures of cobalamin and its derivatives.

HOCbl and AdoCbl are the most frequent forms found in meats, while MeCbl is usually found in dairy products. AdoCbl and MeCbl are cofactors in several enzymes which catalyse complex molecular transformations which involve the breakage of the Co–C bond as the first step [1, 2]. For example, AdoCbl-dependent enzymes catalyse rearrangement reactions which are facilitated by radical intermediates [1], while MeCbl is a cofactor which catalyses the intermolecular methyl (CH_3) transfer reactions [3]. CNCbl is inactive in mammalian cells. In the mitochondria, the AdoCbl serves as a coenzyme of the methylmalonyl–CoA mutase. Nevertheless, vitamin B_{12} can be used after it has been converted into activating forms (i.e. AdoCbl or MeCbl). Figure 9.2 shows the steps necessary to convert each form of vitamin B_{12}.

MeCbl is the most effective form of vitamin B_{12} in subcellular organelles of neurons. Thus, MeCbl may offer excellent therapy for nervous disorders via effective local or systemic delivery. As a supportive agent, MeCbl can treat Alzheimer's disease syndromes [4] and vitamin B_{12} deficiency [5].

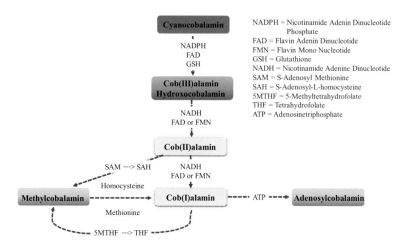

Figure 9.2 Conversion steps of each form of vitamin B_{12} (Source: www.vitaminb12.de).

9.1 Vitamin B_{12} as an Active Ingredient of Supplements

The synthetic hydroxocobalamin (HOCbl) and cyanocobalamin (CNCbl) forms have been used traditionally as vitamin B_{12} shots. The synthetic CNCbl and HOCbl forms are commonly used for oral supplements, such as capsules and tablets. Adenosylcobalamin (AdoCbl) and methylcobalamin (MeCbl) are the readily useable bioactive forms of vitamin B_{12}; however, they are unstable outside the body because of their photosensitivity, which makes them difficult to produce. On the other hand, AdoCbl and MeCbl forms have become more readily available as supplements because of their important therapeutic value.

9.2 Efficacy Spectrum of Bioactive Vitamin B_{12} Forms

9.2.1 Cyanocobalamin vs. Hydroxocobalamin

CNCbl has a considerably poorer sustained release and absorption rate compared to HOCbl. Therefore, HOCbl is more frequently preferred when administering injections. This is attributed to the less metabolic route needed when breaking down HOCbl as compared to CNCbl. Moreover, HOCbl shows no danger of cyanide poisoning; therefore, HOCbl is used as cyanide detoxification. CNCbl commonly results in smoke inhalation/heavy smoking in the human body with a normal diet. Therefore, smokers are advised not to take CNCbl but other vitamin B_{12} forms. HOCbl also efficiently reduces nitric oxide, which is responsible for causing oxidative stress.

9.2.2 Cyanocobalamin vs. Methylcobalamin

MeCbl-based supplements are rapidly gaining popularity over CNCbl in the market. MeCbl contains a methyl group, while CNCbl has a cyanide group. Although the level of cyanide in the vitamin B_{12} supplement is too small to be toxic, it is still important to remove cyanide levels from the human body. Since the human body needs the methyl compound to function properly, it is essential to convert any CNCbl supplement into MeCbl as soon as possible. The human body can use MeCbl directly without the need for conversion as compared to CNCbl [6]. Moreover, MeCbl shows better cellular absorption compared to CNCbl. When a high oral dose of CNCbl is taken, large quantities remain unused and are passed out with the urine, while MeCbl has been proven to increase the pivotal cellular levels of vitamin B_{12} [6]. MeCbl has been shown to significantly increase the survival rate of mice with cancer, while CNCbl shows little or no effect [7]. This was ascribed to the highly important S-adenosylmethionine, which was regenerated during epigenetic processes. MeCbl is also superior in the treatment of sleep disorders because it encourages melatonin synthesis.

9.2.3 Exercises

1. What is vitamin B_{12} and why do we need it?
2. Where does it come from?
3. Who is at risk for vitamin B_{12} deficiency?
4. What are the best sources for vitamin B_{12}?
5. Are animal foods a good source of vitamin B_{12}?
6. What are the symptoms of vitamin B_{12} deficiency?

7. What happens if vitamin B_{12} deficiency is overlooked or ignored?
8. What are the four types of vitamin B_{12}?
9. Which type of vitamin B_{12} is suitable?
10. What is the best type of vitamin B_{12}?
11. What is the difference between CNCbl and HOCbl?
12. What makes MeCbl a superior health supplement compared to CNCbl?
13. What are the benefits of a vitamin B_{12} supplement?

9.3   Methylcobalamin

MeCbl is a cofactor of methionine synthase, an enzyme which transfers CH_3 groups to homocysteine to restore methionine. MeCbl is a naturally occurring, bioactive coenzyme form of vitamin B_{12}. Thus, our body can use it directly without going through any metabolic steps to make it body-friendly. Therefore, MeCbl is among the two bioactive coenzyme forms of vitamin B_{12}, which our body really needs. MeCbl is present in foods, such as cheese and milk. Only AdoCbl and MeCbl may have a direct positive effect on our health. However, all other forms of vitamin B_{12} must initially be converted into AdoCbl or MeCbl before they can become an active coenzyme in our bodies. In the body, MeCbl is normally found in the central nervous system and cells. MeCbl differs from CNCbl since the cyano (CN) group at the Co is substituted by a methyl (CH_3) group [8]. MeCbl can be obtained as a bright-red crystal with an octahedral cobalt (III) centre [9]. Moreover, MeCbl is a rare compound, which contains a metal–alkyl bond. MeCbl is equal physiologically to vitamin B_{12} and can treat or prevent pernicious anaemia rising from vitamin B_{12} deficiency. MeCbl is also used as an initial treatment of amyotrophic lateral sclerosis, in addition to the treatment of diabetic neuropathy and peripheral neuropathy [10]. MeCbl cannot be used as a direct cofactor when ingested; however, it is initially converted into cob(II)alamin by homocystinuria. Subsequently, cob(II)alamin is then transformed into MeCbl and AdoCbl, which can be used as cofactors [11–13].

MeCbl works directly within the cells, and it is responsible for the reactivation of folic acid. Thus, folic acid remains unusable without MeCbl and cannot have a positive effect on the body. This can cause genetic errors during cell division, nerve damage and anaemia. MeCbl can liberate the dangerous amino acid (i.e. homocysteine) which endangers blood vessels and induces cardiovascular issues. The corresponding methionine, which is a precursor of S-adenosylmethionine, plays a crucial part in the synthesis of neurotransmitters, protection of nerves and regulation of genes and enzymes. A deficiency in S-adenosylmethionine causes difficulty in nerve disorders, increased risk of a variety of diseases and mood changes. MeCbl supplementation can help in improving sleep–wake cycles, normalising circadian rhythms, enhancing light sensitivity and modulating melatonin secretion. MeCbl also enhances heart rate variability and sympathetic nervous system function via its association with melatonin synthesis and light entrainment.

During a single reaction, MeCbl can:

1. Reactivate the folic acid
2. Break down the dangerous homocysteine
3. Create a precursor of S-adenosylmethionine

9.3.1 Mechanisms Underlying the Analgesic Action of MeCbl

Vitamin B_{12} has been used to increase the effectiveness of 5-hydroxytryptamine and noradrenaline in the inhibitory nociceptive system [14]. MeCbl exerts neuropathic ache in diabetics patient via its neuroprotective and neurosynthesis actions [15]. Nonetheless, the analgesic mechanism of MeCbl remained elusive until now.

9.3.1.1 Enhancing the nerve conduction velocity

Studies have shown that high doses of MeCbl enhance nerve conduction in streptozotocin diabetic rats [16] and patients with experimental acrylamide neuropathy [17] and diabetic neuropathy [18]. Histological and morphological evidence has confirmed that continuous use of MeCbl promotes regeneration and myelin synthesis, as well as enhancing the nerve neuronal function and conduction velocity in peripheral neuropathy of myelin [19].

9.3.1.2 Improving the rejuvenation of wounded nerves

MeCbl was able to recover injured nerves by introducing radioactive leucine into the protein segment of the rumpled sciatic nerves in vivo [20]. In the sciatic nerve injury and experimental acrylamide neuropathy simulations, the number of rejuvenations of motor fibres revealed much improvement with high doses of MeCbl [17] Moreover, the collective use of pyridoxal 5′-phosphate, MeCbl and L-methylfolate enhanced the calf muscle surface neural density [21].

9.3.1.3 Constraining ectopic spontaneous release

Ectopic spontaneous release is anticipated to initiate allodynia, hyperalgesia and spontaneous pains [22]. MeCbl has been reported to suppress the ectopic fringe caused by chemical material in a dog dorsal root [23]. MeCbl evidently restrained the ectopic spontaneous discharges of dorsal root ganglion neurons in dorsal root ganglion rats, as well as inhibiting peripheral pain signals [4].

9.3.2 Exercises

1. What is MeCbl and why do you need it?
2. How does MeCbl work?
3. What are the special effects of MeCbl?
4. Is MeCbl natural?
5. Who should supplement with MeCbl?
6. Do people with methylation defect take the MeCbl form of vitamin B_{12}?

9.4 Adenosylcobalamin

Besides HOCbl, AdoCbl is a naturally occurring form of vitamin B_{12} commonly present in foods [24]. Alongside MeCbl, AdoCbl is one of the two forms of a bioactive coenzyme which the human body needs. AdoCbl is a cofactor for the metabolism of enzymes in bacteria, humans and other mammals [25]. AdoCbl is mostly used in the mitochondria, which act as the engine room of the cells. AdoCbl acts within the mitochondria as a chemical building block of the enzyme methylmalonyl-CoA mutase, which is converted to succinyl-CoA, a central metabolic cycle for the production of energy [26, 27]. Moreover, AdoCbl is also involved in the provision of vital hormones and amino acids, such as thymine, methionine, threonine, isoleucine and valine. AdoCbl as a cofactor for enzymes can undergo elimination reactions via radical-based chemistry, as well as catalyse carbon skeleton rearrangements [28]. AdoCbl has been used very effectively for many years by several naturopaths and doctors in the form of AdoCbl capsules, drops and vials, which are available in several pharmaceutical shops. Thus, AdoCbl is useful in combating hepatitis, liver damage, chronic tiredness and exhaustion, weight loss and anorexia, muscle weakness and fibromyalgia [29, 30].

AdoCbl contains a Co–C bond and can be used as a light sensor by the light-dependent transcription factor [31]. The photochemistry of AdoCbl has been extensively studied [32]. The exposure of AdoCbl to <550 nm light induces a homolytic cleavage of the Co–C bonds [32], which generates a five-coordinate cob(II)alamin as well as the 5′-deoxyadenosyl radical. This cleavage is harnessed by a photoreceptor protein (CarH). Under aerobic conditions, the 5′-deoxyadenosyl radical quickly combines with molecular oxygen (O_2) to form 5′-peroxyadenosine, which then breaks down to produce adenosine-5′-aldehyde, with adenine and adenosine as minor products (Scheme 9.1) [33].

The ultraviolet (UV)-visible spectrum of the CarH free dark state is equivalent to the free AdoCbl [34]. In the presence of oxygen, CarH-bound cobalamin (Cbl) has a Co(III) oxidation state [34]. However, in the absence of oxygen, the oxidation state of Cbl is Co(II), as shown by electron spin resonance spectroscopy and UV-visible spectroscopy [35]. Under anaerobic photolysis, exposure of CarH-bound Cbl with Co(II) generates cob(II) and 5′,8-cycloadenosine as the major products [36]. AdoCbl can serve as a cofactor for CarH, which controls the expression of DNA coding for the transcription of proteins required for the fabrication of carotenes using nonphotosynthetic bacteria [25]. The UV-visible spectroscopic and Co–C bond photolysis investigation reveals that AdoCbl is not much altered in the enzyme–coenzyme–substrate ternary complex [37]. In addition, substrate binding cannot change the protein to a structural state, which can quickly stabilise radical pair generation [37]. The underlying microscopic mechanism, which constitutes the design of favourable binding energy between the 5′-deoxyadenosyl radical and

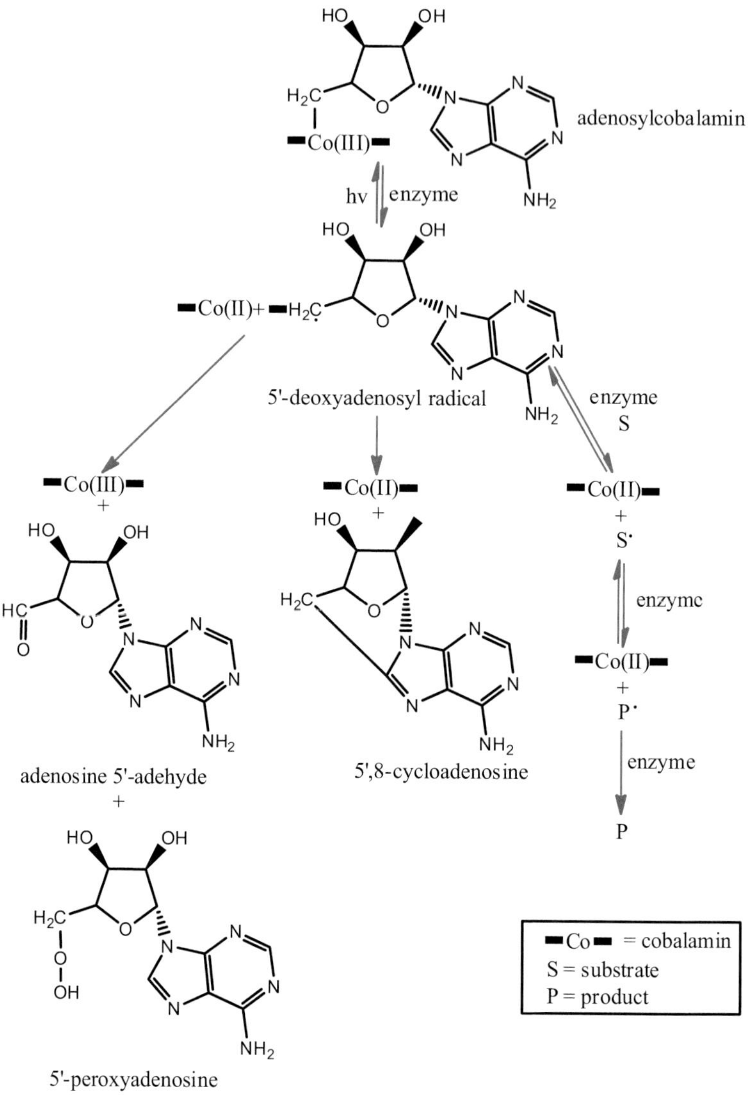

126 | Vitamin B₁₂ Derivatives

Scheme 9.1 Homolysis of the Co–C bond of adenosylcobalamin.

the protein, has also been proposed by modelling and theory [38]. Spectroscopic studies using resonance Raman, magnetic circular dichroism (MCD) and UV-visible absorption have revealed that AdoCbl is not much altered in the presence of substrate analogues or in the MCM holoenzyme compared to the solution form [39]. The structure of cob(II)alamin, which is the cleavage product, is also not much affected by protein [40]. The lack of ground-state Co–C bond activation by the enzyme was established from the infrared [41] and picosecond optical [42] spectroscopic investigations. Obviously, nuclear magnetic resonance (NMR) spectroscopy and liquid chromatography–mass spectrometry (LC-MS) studies have shown that the AdoCbl-bound CarH under both aerobic and anaerobic conditions revealed 4′,5′-anhydroadenosine as the only organic photolysis product [35]. Moreover, 4′,5′-anhydroadenosine has been detected in the thermolysis of AdoCbl in glycerol [43], and this might offer a model for the photolysis of CarH-bound AdoCbl. The 5′-deoxyadenosyl radical, which was produced by homolytic fission and Co(II), would undergo a β-elimination reaction to generate HOCbl and 4′,5′-anhydroadenosine [43]. The HOCbl then quickly breaks down to form a hydrogen and Co(II) (Scheme 9.2) [43].

Jost and coworkers [35] further proposed the CarH photolysis mechanism (see Scheme 9.3, paths 1 and 2) on the basis of the results presented by Garr and Finke [43].

The CarH-bound AdoCbl initially goes through photolysis to produce a 5′-deoxyadenosyl radical and Co(II) via homolytic fission of the Co–C bond (see path 1 of Scheme 9.3). Besides the thermolysis of adenosylcobinamide and AdoCbl [43], homolytic fission followed by a radical-mediated β-elimination reaction has been established in alkylcobinamides and alkylcobalamins [44]. The formation of 4′,5′-anhydroadenosine as the organic product of CarH photolysis may signify a suitable mechanism to ensure that the reactive 5′-deoxyadenosyl radical is not discharged [35]. Path 2 of Scheme 9.3 involves the preliminary heterolytic breaking of the Co–C bond to form a 5′-deoxyadenosyl anion and Co(III), followed by the β-elimination reaction to generate HOCbl and 4′,5′-anhydroadenosine [35]. Kutta and coworkers [45] proposed a different path 2, where heterolysis of the Co–C bond gave a 5′-deoxyadenosyl anion, as well as a five-coordinated positively charged Co(III) or HOCbl as an intermediate to give a cob(II)alamin and 4′,5′-anhydroadenosine. Path 3 of Scheme 9.3 involves a concerted β-elimination reaction through the transfer of a hydride ion to form 4′,5′-anhydroadenosine and HOCbl.

128 | Vitamin B₁₂ Derivatives

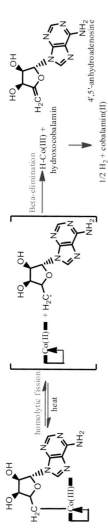

Scheme 9.2 Thermolysis pathway of adenosylcobalamin in glycerol, which was formed via homolytic fission followed by β-elimination [25].

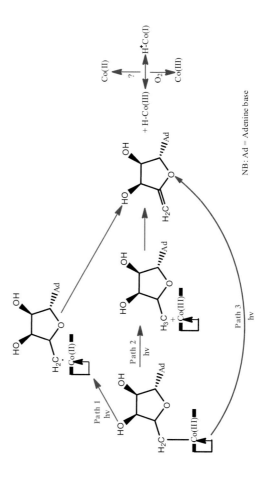

Scheme 9.3 Proposed pathway for CarH [25].

The wild-type CarH forms a stable complex with Cbl after photolysis has occurred, while the Cbl moiety binds strongly to the light-state CarH [34]. Similarly, the Cbl-dependent light-sensing protein AerR in *Rhodobacter capsulatus* forms a stable complex with Cbl [46]. This complex comprises Cbl bound to two histidines from the protein at both bottom and top positions [46]. Nonetheless, this type of coordination of histidine is contentious since it has not been perceived for free Cbl [47]. The equilibrium constant of the coordination of Co(III) to the first histidine (log K_2 = 14.30) was favourable; however, the coordination of Co(III) to the second histidine was much more difficult (log K_2 < –1) [47]. This indicates that the spectrum of the bis histidine complex cannot be perceived [47]. Nevertheless, the UV-visible spectra of Cbl with dbzm in the lower position and imidazole or histidine in the upper position are almost identical [47]. The UV-visible spectrum of a bis–imidazole complex of Cbl was perceived as log K_1 = 4.59 and log K_2 = 0.6 [47]. The UV-visible spectrum of the light-state CarH protein was indistinguishable from that of the Co(III)–Cbl complex with two imidazole ligands binding via the N atoms in the lower and upper positions [35]. This was in agreement with the replacement of Cbl with two histidines of the protein [19].

9.4.1 Exercises

1. What is AdoCbl?
2. What are the uses of AdoCbl?
3. How exactly is the Co–C bond in CarH-bound AdoCbl broken?
4. What are the products of photolysis of CarH-bound AdoCbl?
5. How is the Co(III) in the light-state CarH protein bonded to the second histidine (His 132) on the protein?

9.5 Cyanocobalamin

CNCbl is a synthetic form of vitamin B_{12}. Generally, CNCbl is a form of vitamin B_{12} since the human body can transform CNCbl to other active forms of vitamin B_{12} [48]. CNCbl is normally used after surgical removal of all or part of the intestine or stomach, and this ensures suitable serum levels of vitamin B_{12}. CNCbl is used in the treatment of kidney disease, liver disease, haemorrhage, thyrotoxicosis, pernicious anaemia and malignancy. CNCbl is used to carry out the Schilling test to examine how the body can absorb vitamin B_{12}. Besides it importance, CNCbl injection can cause allergic reactions, such as diarrhoea; extreme thirst; swelling of the feet, ankles, lower legs, hands and arms; redness of the face; hives; and difficulty in breathing. However, less serious side effects include rash, itching, leg pain, dizziness and headache. Treatment of megaloblastic anaemia builds the possibility of hypokalaemia owing to the increased cellular uptake of potassium upon anaemia resolution and red blood cell production.

9.5.1 Chemical Reactions

Usually, cobalt (Co) is in the trivalent state (i.e. Co(III)) in Cbls. Nonetheless, under reducing conditions, the Co centre is reduced to either Co(II) or Co(I), which are represented as B_{12s} and B_{12r} for super-reduced and reduced, respectively. B_{12s} and B_{12r} can be fabricated from CNCbl through controlled chemical or potential reduction using sodium borohydride and zinc in acetic acid or in alkaline solution. Both B_{12s} and B_{12r} are stable under oxygen-free conditions. B_{12s} appears purple under artificial light and bluish-green under natural daylight, while B_{12r} appears orange-brown in solution [49]. In aqueous solution, B_{12s} is among the most suitable nucleophilic species. This property permits the appropriate fabrication of Cbl analogues with different substituents through a nucleophilic attack on the vinyl and alkyl halides [49]. In particular, CNCbl is transformed to its analogue Cbls through reduction to B_{12s}. Subsequently, alkyne, alkene, acyl halides and alkyl halides were added. The major hindrance in the synthesis of B_{12} coenzyme analogues is a steric hindrance. For instance, no reaction can occur between B_{12s} and neopentyl chloride, while the secondary alkyl halide analogues are too unstable to be inaccessible [49]. This outcome can be ascribed to the strong coordination between the central C atom and benzimidazole. The trans effect controls the polarisability of the Co–C bond formed. Nonetheless, after the benzimidazole is separated from Co by quarterisation with CH_3I, it is substituted by hydroxyl ions or H_2O. Subsequently, several secondary alkyl halides are easily bound by the modified B_{12s} to form a corresponding stable Cbl analogue [50]. The products are commonly extracted and purified by column chromatography or the phenol-methylene chloride extraction approach [49]. Cbl analogues prepared by the above approach comprise the naturally occurring coenzymes cobamamide, MeCbl, as well as other Cbls which do not occur naturally (i.e. cyclohexylcobalamin, carboxymethylcobalamin and vinylcobalamin) [49].

Recently CNCbl has received increasing criticism, such as lack of prolonged release, methyl group raiders, utilisation difficulties, bioavailability, build-up in cells and toxicity [51–53].

9.5.2 Exercises

1. What is CNCbl?
2. Who should use CNCbl?
3. Is the CNCbl form of vitamin B_{12} safe?
4. What happens when you take too much CNCbl?
5. What are the effects of CNCbl?

9.6 Hydroxocobalamin

HOCbl, also known as hydroxycobalamin, is a natural form of vitamin B_{12}. HOCbl is produced by most microorganisms and is one of the most common vitamin B_{12} forms found in natural food sources [24]. HOCbl has received considerable interest since the photolysis of HOCbl in the presence of oxygen was utilised to cleave plasmid DNA [54].

9.6.1 Special Effects of Hydroxocobalamin

9.6.1.1 Long-lasting effects and sustained release

HOCbl binds to the body's transport molecules and circulates much longer in the blood compared to the other vitamin B_{12} forms. This ensures a balanced and long-lasting supply of vitamin B_{12} [55]. HOCbl also acts as a suitable sustained release, and this ensures that the body's vitamin B_{12} store is optimally topped up, as well as ensuring

132 | Vitamin B₁₂ Derivatives

an even supply of vitamin B_{12} for the cells. This protects the body during periods of difficulty or stress.

9.6.1.2 Detoxing and quitting smoking

Moreover, HOCbl carries out other special effects, such as disease preventative and detox effects before conversion to its coenzyme forms. This is because HOCbl is a superb cyanide catcher and can treat smoke poisoning [56]. Therefore, the active ingredient may be an excellent tool to aid a person who wants to quit smoking, as well as detoxifying the human body.

9.6.1.3 Blocking nitrosative stress

HOCbl can also block nitric oxide radicals, and therefore, it is an excellent approach for the advancement of nitrosative stress, which causes a wide variety of diseases.

9.6.1.4 Hydroxocobalamin supplements: pills and capsules

When the amount of absorbed HOCbl present in the oral supplement exceeds its limits in the intestine, the long-lasting effects and outstanding resorption of HOCbl active ingredients come into play [57].

Application of hydroxyl radicals, which are generated photochemically through the homolytic cleavage of the Co−OH bond, provide several benefits compared to the Fenton reaction using FeII ethylenediaminetetraacetic acid (EDTA) and H_2O_2. Moreover, HOCbl has an advantage of controlling the intracellular temporal by light-dependent photo-initiated reactions as compared to chemical methods, where initiation and termination of the radical reactions cannot be exactly contained [58]. Anaerobic photolysis with a radical scavenger, such as sorbitol or sodium benzoate, shows no measurable photolysis at a wavelength of >350 nm. However, photolysis to generate cob(II)alamin is readily observed following excitation at a wavelength of 253 nm.

9.6.2 Exercises

1. What is HOCbl?
2. What are the special effects of HOCbl?

3. What should be avoided while taking HOCbl**?**
4. What are the possible side effects of HOCbl**?**

References

1. E. N. G. Marsh, G. D. R. Meléndez, Adenosylcobalamin enzymes: theory and experiment begin to converge, *Biochim. Biophys. Acta, Proteins Proteomics*, **1824** (2012) 1154–1164.

2. M. L. Ludwig, R. G. Matthews, Structure-based perspectives on B_{12}-dependent enzymes, *Annu. Rev. Biochem.*, **66** (1997) 269–313.

3. R. G. Matthews, M. Koutmos, S. Datta, Cobalamin-dependent and cobamide-dependent methyltransferases, *Curr. Opin. Struct. Biol.*, **18** (2008) 658–666.

4. M. Zhang, W. Han, S. Hu, H. Xu, Methylcobalamin: a potential vitamin of pain killer, *Neural Plast.*, **2013** (2013) 1–6.

5. A. McCaddon, P. R. Hudson, L-methylfolate, methylcobalamin, and N-acetylcysteine in the treatment of Alzheimer's disease-related cognitive decline, *CNS Spectr.*, **15** (2010) 2–5.

6. K. Okuda, K. Yashima, T. Kitazaki, I. Takara, Intestinal absorption and concurrent chemical changes of methylcobalamin, *Transl. Res.*, **81** (1973) 557–567.

7. C. S. Tsao, K. Myashita, Influence of cobalamin on the survival of mice bearing ascites tumor, *Pathobiology*, **61** (1993) 104–108.

8. L. McDowell, *Vitamins in Animal and Human Nutrition*, 2nd ed., Iowa State University Press, Ames, Iowa, 2000.

9. D. Dophin, [205] Preparation of the reduced forms of vitamin B_{12} and of some analogs of the vitamin B_{12} coenzyme containing a cobalt-carbon bond, *Methods in Enzymol.*, **18**(Part C) (1971) 34–52.

10. L. A. Smolin, M. B. Grosvenor, *Nutrition: Science and Applications*, 1st ed., Saunders College Publishing, 1994.

11. J. Kim, L. Hannibal, C. Gherasim, D. W. Jacobsen, R. Banerjee, A human vitamin B_{12} trafficking protein uses glutathione transferase activity for processing alkylcobalamins, *J. Biol. Chem.*, **284** (2009) 33418–33424.

12. L. Hannibal, J. Kim, N. E. Brasch, S. Wang, D. S. Rosenblatt, R. Banerjee, D. W. Jacobsen, Processing of alkylcobalamins in mammalian cells: a role for the MMACHC (cblC) gene product, *Mol. Genet. Metab.*, **97** (2009) 260–266.

13. D. S. Froese, R. A. Gravel, Genetic disorders of vitamin B_{12} metabolism: eight complementation groups-eight genes, *Expert Rev. Mol. Med.*, **12** (2010) 1–20.

14. I. Jurna, Analgesic and analgesia-potentiating action of B vitamins, *Schmerz*, **12** (1998) 136–141.

15. Y. Sun, M.-S. Lai, C.-J. Lu, Effectiveness of vitamin B_{12} on diabetic neuropathy: systematic review of clinical controlled trials, *Acta Neurol. Taiwan*, **14** (2005) 48–54.

16. M. Sonobe, H. Yasuda, I. Hatanaka, M. Terada, M. Yamashita, R. Kikkawa, Y. Shigeta, Methylcobalamin improves nerve conduction in streptozotocin-diabetic rats without affecting sorbitol and myo-inositol contents of sciatic nerve, *Horm. Metab. Res.*, **20** (1988) 717–718.

17. T. Watanabe, R. Kaji, N. Oka, W. Bara, J. Kimura, Ultra-high dose methylcobalamin promotes nerve regeneration in experimental acrylamide neuropathy, *J. Neurol. Sci.*, **122** (1994) 140–143.

18. G. Devathasan, W. Teo, A. Mylvaganam, Methylcobalamin ($CH_3–B_{12}$; methycobal) in chronic diabetic neuropathy. A double blind clinical and electrophysiological study, *Clin. Trials J.*, **23** (1986) 130–140.

19. K. Okada, H. Tanaka, K. Temporin, M. Okamoto, Y. Kuroda, H. Moritomo, T. Murase, H. Yoshikawa, Methylcobalamin increases Erk1/2 and Akt activities through the methylation cycle and promotes nerve regeneration in a rat sciatic nerve injury model, *Exp. Neurol.*, **222** (2010) 191–203.

20. K. Yamatsu, Y. Yamanishi, T. Kaneko, I. Ohkawa, Pharmacological studies on degeneration and regeneration of the peripheral nerves. Effects of methylcobalamin on mitosis of Schwann cells and incorporation of labeled amino acid into protein fractions of crushed sciatic nerve in rats, *Nihon Yakurigaku Zasshi*, **72** (1976) 269–278.

21. A. Jacobs, D. Cheng, Management of diabetic small-fiber neuropathy with combination L-methylfolate, methylcobalamin, and pyridoxal 5′-phosphate, *Rev. Neurol. Dis.*, **8** (2010) 39–47.

22. S. R. Chaplan, H.-Q. Guo, D. H. Lee, L. Luo, C. Liu, C. Kuei, A. A. Velumian, M. P. Butler, S. M. Brown, A. E. Dubin, Neuronal hyperpolarization-activated pacemaker channels drive neuropathic pain, *J. Neurosci.*, **23** (2003) 1169–1178.

23. Y. Atsuta, T. Iwahara, O. Sugawara, T. Muramoto, T. Watakabe, Y. Takemisu, The study of generating and suppressive factors of ectopic firing in the lumbar dorsal root using an *in vivo* model, *Clin. Orthop.*, **29** (1994) 441–446.

24. J. Farquharson, J. Adams, The forms of vitamin B_{12} in foods, *Br. J. Nutr.*, **36** (1976) 127–136.

25. S. M. Chemaly, New light on vitamin B_{12}: the adenosylcobalamin-dependent photoreceptor protein CarH, *S. Afr. J. Sci.*, **112** (2016) 1–9.

26. E. Marsh, Coenzyme B_{12} (cobalamin)-dependent enzymes, *Essays Biochem.*, **34** (1999) 139–154.

27. H. G. Wood, R. W. Kellermeyer, R. Stjernholm, S. Allen, Metabolism of methylmalonyl-CoA and the role of biotin and B_{12} coenzymes, *Ann. N. Y. Acad. Sci.*, **112** (1964) 661–679.

28. L. Mander, H.-W. Liu, *Comprehensive Natural Products II: Chemistry and Biology*, Newnes, Italy, 2010.

29. M. Korkina, G. Korchak, D. Medvedev, Clinico-experimental substantiation of the use of carnitine and cobalamin in the treatment of anorexia nervosa, *Zh. Nevropatol. Psikhiatr. Im. S S Korsakova*, **89** (1989) 82–87.

30. S. Iwarson, J. Lindberg, Coenzyme-B_{12} therapy in acute viral hepatitis, *Scand. J. Infect. Dis.*, **9** (1977) 157–158.

31. J. M. Ortiz-Guerrero, M. C. Polanco, F. J. Murillo, S. Padmanabhan, M. Elías-Arnanz, Light-dependent gene regulation by a coenzyme B_{12}-based photoreceptor, *Proc. Natl. Acad. Sci.*, **108** (2011) 7565–7570.

32. E. Chen, M. R. Chance, Nanosecond transient absorption spectroscopy of coenzyme B_{12}. Quantum yields and spectral dynamics, *J. Biol. Chem.*, **265** (1990) 12987–12994.

33. P. A. Schwartz, P. A. Frey, 5′-Peroxyadenosine and 5′-peroxyadenosylcobalamin as intermediates in the aerobic photolysis of adenosylcobalamin, *Biochemistry*, **46** (2007) 7284–7292.

34. M. Jost, J. Fernández-Zapata, M. C. Polanco, J. M. Ortiz-Guerrero, P. Y.-T. Chen, G. Kang, S. Padmanabhan, M. Elías-Arnanz, C. L. Drennan, Structural basis for gene regulation by a B_{12}-dependent photoreceptor, *Nature*, **526** (2015) 536.

35. M. Jost, J. H. Simpson, C. L. Drennan, The transcription factor CarH safeguards use of adenosylcobalamin as a light sensor by altering the photolysis products, *Biochemistry*, **54** (2015) 3231–3234.

36. P. Law, J. Wood, The photolysis of 5′-deoxyadenosylcobalamin under anaerobic conditions, *Biochim. Biophys. Acta, Nucleic Acids Protein Synth.*, **331** (1973) 451–454.

37. W. D. Robertson, M. Wang, K. Warncke, Characterization of protein contributions to cobalt-carbon bond cleavage catalysis in

adenosylcobalamin-dependent ethanolamine ammonia-lyase by using photolysis in the ternary complex, *J. Am. Chem. Soc.*, **133** (2011) 6968–6977.

38. D. Bucher, G. M. Sandala, B. Durbeej, L. Radom, D. M. Smith, The elusive 5'-deoxyadenosyl radical in coenzyme-B_{12}-mediated reactions, *J. Am. Chem. Soc.*, **134** (2012) 1591–1599.

39. A. J. Brooks, M. Vlasie, R. Banerjee, T. C. Brunold, Spectroscopic and computational studies on the adenosylcobalamin-dependent methylmalonyl-CoA mutase: evaluation of enzymatic contributions to Co–C bond activation in the Co^{3+} ground state, *J. Am. Chem. Soc.*, **126** (2004) 8167–8180.

40. A. J. Brooks, M. Vlasie, R. Banerjee, T. C. Brunold, Co–C bond activation in methylmalonyl-CoA mutase by stabilization of the post-homolysis product Co^{2+} cobalamin, *J. Am. Chem. Soc.*, **127** (2005) 16522–16528.

41. S. Dong, R. Padmakumar, R. Banerjee, T. G. Spiro, Co–C bond activation in B_{12}-dependent enzymes: cryogenic resonance raman studies of methylmalonyl-coenzyme a mutase, *J. Am. Chem. Soc.*, **121** (1999) 7063–7070.

42. R. J. Sension, D. A. Harris, A. Stickrath, A. G. Cole, C. C. Fox, E. N. G. Marsh, Time-resolved measurements of the photolysis and recombination of adenosylcobalamin bound to glutamate mutase, *J. Phys. Chem. B*, **109** (2005) 18146–18152.

43. C. D. Garr, R. G. Finke, Adocobalamin (AdoCbl or coenzyme B_{12}) cobalt-carbon bond homolysis radical-cage effects: product, kinetic, mechanistic, and cage efficiency factor (Fc) studies, plus the possibility that coenzyme B_{12}-dependent enzymes function as "ultimate radical cages" and "ultimate radical traps", *Inorg. Chem.*, **32** (1993) 4414–4421.

44. D. A. Baldwin, E. A. Betterton, S. M. Chemaly, J. M. Pratt, The chemistry of vitamin B_{12}. Part 25. Mechanism of the β-elimination of olefins from alkylcorrinoids; evidence for an initial homolytic fission of the Co–C bond, *Dalton Trans.*, (1985) 1613–1618.

45. R. J. Kutta, S. J. Hardman, L. O. Johannissen, B. Bellina, H. L. Messiha, J. M. Ortiz-Guerrero, M. Elías-Arnanz, S. Padmanabhan, P. Barran, N. S. Scrutton, The photochemical mechanism of a B_{12}-dependent photoreceptor protein, *Nat. Commun.*, **6** (2015) 1–11.

46. Z. Cheng, K. Li, L. A. Hammad, J. A. Karty, C. E. Bauer, Vitamin B_{12} regulates photosystem gene expression via the CrtJ antirepressor AerR in Rhodobacter capsulatus, *Mol. Microbiol.*, **91** (2014) 649–664.

47. H. M. Marques, J. H. Marsh, J. R. Mellor, O. Q. Munro, The coordination of imidazole and its derivatives by aquocobalamin, *Inorg. Chim. Acta*, **170** (1990) 259–269.

48. E. V. Quadros, Advances in the understanding of cobalamin assimilation and metabolism, *Br. J. Haematol.*, **148** (2010) 195–204.

49. D. Dolphin, Preparation of the reduced forms of vitamin B_{12} and of some analogs of the vitamin B_{12} coenzyme containing a cobalt-carbon bond, *Methods Enzymol.*, **18** (1971) 34–52.

50. J. D. Brodie, On the mechanism of catalysis by vitamin B_{12}, *Proc. Natl. Acad. Sci.*, **62** (1969) 461–467.

51. P. Gimsing, E. Hippe, I. Helleberg-Rasmussen, M. Moesgaard, J. L. Nielsen, P. Bastrup-Madsen, R. Berlin, T. Hansen, Cobalamin forms in plasma and tissue during treatment of vitamin B_{12} deficiency, *Eur. J. Haematol.*, **29** (1982) 311–318.

52. E. Pezacka, R. Green, D. W. Jacobsen, Glutathionylcobalamin as an intermediate in the formation of cobalamin coenzymes, *Biochem. Biophys. Res. Commun.*, **169** (1990) 443–450.

53. H. C. Andersson, E. Shapira, Biochemical and clinical response to hydroxocobalamin versus cyanocobalamin treatment in patients with methylmalonic acidemia and homocystinuria (cblC), *J. Pediatr.*, **132** (1998) 121–124.

54. T. A. Shell, D. S. Lawrence, A new trick (hydroxyl radical generation) for an old vitamin (B_{12}), *J. Am. Chem. Soc.*, **133** (2011) 2148–2150.

55. K. Boddy, P. King, L. Mervyn, A. Macleod, J. Adams, Retention of cyanocobalamin, hydroxocobalamin, and coenzyme B_{12} after parenteral administration, *Lancet*, **292** (1968) 710–712.

56. G. Shepherd, L. I. Velez, Role of hydroxocobalamin in acute cyanide poisoning, *Ann. Pharmacother.*, **42** (2008) 661–669.

57. C. A. Hall, J. A. Begley, P. D. Green-Colligan, The availability of therapeutic hydroxocobalamin to cells, *Blood*, **63** (1984) 335–341.

58. J. J. Shiang, A. G. Cole, R. J. Sension, K. Hang, Y. Weng, J. S. Trommel, L. G. Marzilli, T. Lian, Ultrafast excited-state dynamics in vitamin B_{12} and related cob (III) alamins, *J. Am. Chem. Soc.*, **128** (2006) 801–808.

Chapter 10

Theoretical Approach

10.1 Mechanism of the S_1 Excited-State Internal Conversion in Vitamin B$_{12}$

Studies using ultrafast transient absorption spectroscopy reveal that the time scale of vitamin B$_{12}$ excited-state dynamic is between femtoseconds and nanoseconds [1]. Therefore, the specific mechanisms of photolysis rely on the form of the substituent group and the environment of the cofactor, for example enzyme or solvent [1]. To check the mechanism for the photochemical production of hydroxyl radicals from HOCbl, broadband femtosecond ultraviolet-visible transient absorption spectroscopy was used to characterise the excited electronic states of HOCbl and the results were compared with time-domain density functional theory (TD-DFT) calculations [2]. An earlier measurement of hydroxocobalamin (HOCbl) was performed in D$_2$O with a mixture of D$_2$OCbl and DOCbl complicating the interpretation [3]. The excited-state lifetime of aquacobalamin (H$_2$OCbl) was substantially shorter than that of HOCbl [4].

The species-associated difference spectra (SADS) can be used to determine the excited-state spectra by adding the appropriate ground-state contribution to the different spectra:

$$A(\lambda) = \Delta A(\lambda) + \alpha A_{GS}(\lambda),$$

Molecular Modelling of Vitamin B$_{12}$ and Its Analogues
Penny Poomani Govender, Francis Opoku, Olaide Olalekan Wahab, and Ephraim Muriithi Kiarii
Copyright © 2022 Jenny Stanford Publishing Pte. Ltd.
ISBN 978-981-4877-58-9 (Hardcover), 978-1-003-21339-0 (eBook)
www.jennystanford.com

where α is the fraction of the ground state excited by the pump pulse [5]. The spectrum of the S_n state was broad, which extend across the full spectral region. The sensitivity of cobalamin (Cbl) spectra to the axial ligation indicated that the S_n state is characterised by significant elongation of the axial bonds, while the S_1 state has a structure comparable to that of the ground state [4]. This was different from the significant displacement found for the S_1 state of cyanocobalamin (CNCbl) [4].

To check the nature of the low-lying excited states of HOCbl, TD-DFT was used to determine the corresponding potential energy surfaces (PESs) [6]. These surfaces were produced using a structural model of HOCbl, employing the BP86/TZVPP level of theory for all the calculations. The energy surfaces analogous to the lowest excited state (S_1) comprise three different electronic states. The association was apparent to the presence of two energy minima, with one at shorter Co–OH and Co–NIm bond lengths and the other at just slightly elongated and much longer Co–OH and Co–NIm bond lengths. The third state appears on the PES at a Co–OH bond length of about 2.5–2.6 Å and within a Co–NIm range of 1.9–2.3 Å.

To achieve a more accurate explanation of the PESs related to the S_1 state, the geometry of the lowest excited state was optimised as a function of the axial bond lengths [7]. General, the PES corresponding to an adiabatic description of S_1 state does not differ much from that generated through vertical excitations. The optimised S_1 axial bond length does not differ much from those of the ground state. This is certainly in sharp difference with CNCbl, where changes are rather significant [8]. To check the photostability of vitamin B_{12}, the internal conversion of the S_1 state was studied by the TD-DFT calculations [7]. The active coordinate of radiationless deactivation was observed as lengthened axial bonds, and this overcomes a 5.0 kcal mol^{-1} energy barrier between the ground (S_0) and the relaxed ligand-to-metal charge transfer (S_1) states.

Although excited-state dynamics of cyanocobalamin have been widely investigated experimentally, there is a partial understanding of the photostability mechanism. Earlier theoretical studies by TD-DFT investigated the nature of the lowest electronic transition and the corresponding PES [9]. The main aim of this chapter is to investigate the electronic spectra of cyanocobalamin and the potential energy curve along the Co–C elongated bond. To obtain a more accurate explanation of the S_1 PES, more dependable energy of the intermediate related to the internal conversion mechanism and the excited-state geometry of cyanocobalamin were studied by means of TD-DFT calculations [10]. The relaxed structural property of the S_1 state was created as a function of both axial Co–NIm and Co–C bond lengths, and a minimum energy crossing point with reference to the S_0 state was then found. This calculation was used to attain mechanisms of S_1-state radiationless deactivation of vitamin B_{12}, which offers novel, in-depth knowledge of the molecular level of the excited-state dynamics of cyanocobalamin, which agree with previous experimental results [11].

The simplified geometrical model indicated as Im–[CoIII(corrin)]–CN$^+$ has been verified to mimic the spectroscopic features and essential structure of vitamin B_{12} precisely [8] using DFT and TD-DFT [12] calculations in an inherent COnductor-like Screening MOdel (COSMO) [13] with the BP86 functional [14, 15] and TZVPP basis set [16], as applied in TURBOMOLE [17]. The dependability of TD-DFT by means of the BP86 functional for the lowest excited states for cyanocobalamin was confirmed from earlier theoretical studies [8].

10.2 Influence of the α (Axial)–Ligand

The distinctive features of coenzyme B_{12} as a naturally occurring organometallic compound with a Co–C α-bond and several model systems comprising a four–nitrogen equatorial model, as well as the axial Co–ligand and Co–C bonds in an octahedral sphere of the Co(III) ion have received much interest [18]. All known vitamin B_{12}–dependent enzyme reactions involve the breaking and making of Co–C bonds [19]. In this perspective, a knowledge of the effects caused by the substitution of the axial ligands and the structure of the equatorial ligand, which can associate with the vital Co–C bond homolysis route in the vitamin B_{12}–dependent enzyme–catalysed reaction. The redox properties, kinetics of axial ligand exchange and relationships between structures have been studied previously [20].

For adenosylcobalamin (AdoCbl), the proposed enzymatic mechanisms consist of the homolytic Co–C bond breaking, while heterolytic cleavage was assumed to occur for methylcobalamin (MeCbl). The interactions of the coenzymes with the peptide chain at the active sites was accountable for the improved Co–C bond homolysis rate (>12 orders) in AdoCbl after it was bonded to the apoenzyme [21]. However, the factors which govern the rate improvement have not yet been completely explained and remain a topic of interest, especially understanding the behaviour of the axial R–Co–L fragment [22]. Moreover, a vital contribution to comprehend the properties of the cofactor from comprehensive vitamin B_{12} models has been studied [23]. This chapter shows fascinating findings with the hydrogen atoms of the alkyl group being replaced by highly electronegative fluorine. In addition, the fluoroalkylcobaloximes obviously showed that the total or partial fluorination of an alkyl group causes a shortening of both the axial Co–N and Co–C bond lengths as compared to the alkylcobaloximes [24]. This result was explained on the basis of the difference in the steric and electronic properties of the alkyl and the corresponding fluoroalkyl group [25]. The fluoroalkyl groups are less influential ligands, thus causing shorter Co–N and Co–C axial bonds as compared to the corresponding alkyl. This was due to the lower electron-donating performance of the fluoroalkyl group with reference to the alkyl analogues. A linear connection between the stability of the Co–C bonds and the electronegativity of the R ligand have been studied with an order of Me < CF_2H < $CFCl_2$ < CF_3 [26]. This relationship was ascribed to the stronger Co–C bond in fluoroalkylcobalamins compared to that in MeCbl.

10.3 Electronic and Steric Effects

Since the axial Co–NB bond lengths are arduous to examine directly by most of the recent accessible experimental methods, first-principles study can be beneficial to gain in-depth knowledge of the nature of the Co–NB binding. The rising attention in modelling the electronic and structural properties of vitamin B_{12} [27] has proved that DFT might be a vital part of coenzyme B_{12} research [28]. Theoretical investigations might be a vital portion of coenzyme B_{12} study. A force field has been designed and used in the past [29] to perform a molecular mechanical calculation on Cbl and has lately been applied to cobaloxime B_{12} forms [30]. Nonetheless, these calculations, although vital for conformational search investigations, may perhaps not be able to explain the underlying mechanisms of coenzyme B_{12}–

supported reaction because the electronic effect cannot be addressed in most force fields calculations. Because of the large size of the Cbl model system, only a few quantum mechanical calculations have been performed on Cbl. In the past, the triaminomethyl cobalt(III)–amide system has been shown as the only historical importance in modern vitamin B_{12} chemistry [31]. Moreover, semi-empirical calculations have been carried out on corrin and cobaloxime models [32], which were initially studied by Zhu and Khostic [33]. These findings have been significant in terms of discussing the balance between the electronic and steric effects which occur in the vitamin B_{12} reaction. In addition, other groups presented the first DFT calculations on vitamin B_{12} forms, which contain the entire corrin ring [34]. The special effects of the different axial substituents on the corrin folding and the Co–C bond lengths were studied using the LACVP** basis set. A less systematic trans-induction and an unsystematic cis-steric effect were found. The corrin structure was inert towards the size of the axial R ligands, which was in contrast to the mechanochemical trigger mechanisms. The highest occupied molecular orbital–lowest unoccupied molecular orbital (HOMO–LUMO) gap energy increases via the steric series, making the corrin less inclined to homolytic cleavage. Moreover, DFT has been used to study the association between the electronic and steric properties of the energetics and trans-axial base of Co–C bond cleavage of several coenzyme forms of vitamin B_{12} [35]. The dissociation energy was observed to be feebly reliant on the trans-axial base and relates to its basicity. Studies have revealed that different exogenous bases stimulate a biological heterolysis differently and the axial base in the free coenzyme has a significant influence on hastening the Co–C bond heterolysis instead of homolysis [36]. Therefore, the explanation of how the kinetic of Co–C bond cleavage is reliant on the steric and electronic properties of the axial base and, thus, the Co–NB bond lengths has been a significant objective in the bioinorganic investigation of vitamin B_{12} coenzymes [36]. To explain how the steric and electronic factors of the trans-axial base affect the Co–NB bond length, 11 different B–[Co^{III}(corrin)]–Rib$^+$ complexes were completely optimised [35]. Among the 11 investigated bases, 2,6-dimethylpyridine (2,6-lutidine or 2,6-Me$_2$Py), 2-methylpyridine (2-picoline or 2-MePy), 1,2,4-trimethylimidazole (1,2,4-Me$_3$Im) and 1,2-dimethylimidazole (1,2-Me$_2$Im) could not form a stable bond with Co (see Table 10.1).

Table 10.1 DFT-optimised Co–NB bond lengths in B–[Co^{III}(corrin)]–Rib$^+$ (Å), together with the corresponding five-coordinate homolysis and heterolysis products, respectively

Structures	pKa	B–[Co^{III}(corrin)]–Rib$^+$	AdoCo(III)Cbi^{a,b}	B–[Co^{II}(corrin)]$^+$	B–[Co^{III}(corrin)]$^{2+}$	Co(IIII)Cbi^a
	5.6	2.341	(2.240)	2.251	1.908	—
	7.2	2.237	—	2.213	1.892	—
	7.3	2.223	2.098 (2.220)	2.212	1.890	2.090

Structures	pKa	B–[Co^{III}(corrin)]–Rib$^+$	AdoCo(III)Cbi^{a,b}	B–[Co^{II}(corrin)]$^+$	B–[Co^{III}(corrin)]$^{2+}$	Co(IIII)Cbi^a
	7.9	NB	2.132 (2.250)	(2.329)	—	2.129
		NB	2.190	NB	NB	—
	5.3	2.335	2.114 (2.230)	2.248	1.917	2.111

(Continued)

Table 10.1 (*Continued*)

Structures	pKa	B–[Co^{III}(corrin)]–Rib$^+$	AdoCo(III)Cbi[a,b]	B–[Co^{II}(corrin)]$^+$	B–[Co^{III}(corrin)]$^{2+}$	Co(III)Cbi[a]
X = CN	1.9	2.396	—	2.264	1.919	—
X = Me	6.0	2.317	—	2.241	1.914	—
X = NMe$_2$	9.7	2.270	—	2.226	1.907	—
(2-Me pyridine)	6.0	NB	2.163 (2.290)	NB	NB	2.150
(2,6-diMe pyridine)	6.6	NB	2.233 (2.370)	NB	NB	2.193

[a]UFF/MM-optimized Co–N(axial base) bond lengths [37].
[b]In parentheses, UFF/MM-optimized Co–N(axial base) bond lengths [38].

The low values calculated for the three sterically hindered bases, 2,6-Me$_2$Py, 2-MePy and 1,2-Me$_2$Im, show that none of them binds to AdoCbi$^+$ at 25°C [35].

10.4   Bond Dissociation Energies

The factors which affect the Co–C bond dissociation energy (BDE) in coenzyme B$_{12}$–dependent enzymes is one of the most vital features of the vitamin B$_{12}$ bioinorganic investigation [35]. A common feature of coenzyme B$_{12}$–dependent enzymes is that the Co–C bonds of vitamin B$_{12}$ are cleaved homolytically to initiate the reaction. Hence, these reactions are started with the cleavage of the organometallic Co–C bond [39]. The calculation of the Co–C BDE has been a subject of extreme experimental study mostly in the Halpern [40] and Finke [41] laboratories, but only lately has this problem been solved quantum mechanically [42]. Theoretically, the energy of the homolytic cleavage of the Co–C$_R$ bonds in the B–[Co^{III}(corrin)]–R$^+$ systems of vitamin B$_{12}$ coenzymes were calculated as

$$BDE = \left(B - [Co^{III}(corrin)] - R^+_{opt}\right) - \left(B - [Co^{II}(corrin)]^+_{opt} - R''_{opt}\right)$$

(10.1)

where 'opt' represent the energy of the optimised structure.

Kinetic studies have revealed that the homolysis of the isolated AdoCbl in an aqueous solution was slow, with a rate of 10^{-9} s^{-1} at 25°C [41]. The Co–C BDE was calculated as 126 ± kJ/mol [41]. Similarly, the equilibrium constant for AdoCbl homolysis was small, with a rate of 7.9 × 10^{-18} M [43]. However, several coenzyme B$_{12}$ forms achieved a catalytic rate of 2–300 s^{-1} ($\Delta G^{\ddagger} \approx$ 60 kJ/mol) [41]. This enzyme appears to increase the rate of the Co–C bond homolysis by an order of magnitude of 12 ± 1 [41] with a lower $\Delta G^{\ddagger}$ of about 60 kJ/mol [43]. Moreover, these enzymes shifted the equilibrium constant towards the homolysis product by an order of 3 × 10^{12} and a BDE of 74 kJ/mol [43]. Earlier theoretical studies have revealed that the B3LYP functional gave too low calculated BDE values [44]. Hence, a Becke–Perdew86 functional [14, 45] for both the calculation of energies at several Co–C bond lengths and geometry optimisation. The Co–C bond strengths and geometries calculated with the Becke–Perdew86 functional were in close agreement with earlier experiment values

[44]. The cleavage of the Co–C bonds was studied by optimising the CoCorImAdo⁺ system, with the Co–C bonds constrained to several distances in a range of 2.0 to 4.0 Å [46]. The Co–C BDE curves in a protein and vacuum are given in Fig. 10.1.

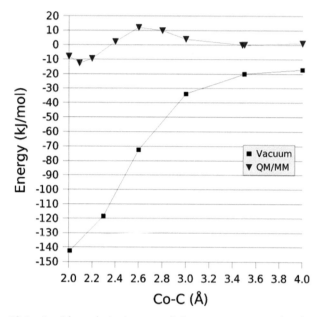

Figure 10.1 Co–C homolytic cleavage of glutamate mutase with reference to the vacuum energies of the CoCorImAdo⁺ model. The reference energy was set at 3.5 Å but at infinite separation in a vacuum [46].

The vacuum curve was similar to previous work reported for the MeCbl and AdoCbl models [27]. However, the total BDE ranges with the quantum mechanics approach used [44]. Remarkably, the vacuum curve gave an energy difference of about 125 kJ/mol in a range of 2.0 to 4.0 Å. However, the isolated product gave a BDE of about 143 kJ/mol.

The influence of protein as the difference between the structures attained at the Co–C bond lengths of 2.0 and 3.5 Å was evaluated [46]. The energy difference was 8 kJ/mol, which favours the Co^{III} state. Moreover, the influence of the protein on the Co–C BDE was 135 kJ/mol (143 − 8 kJ/mol). This effect can be ascribed to the Ado radical not able to dissociate from the enzyme but rather being bound with the corrin ring with hydrogen bonds [41]. The differential stabilisation of the Co^{II} state by the electrostatic interaction with the surrounding protein was observed [46]. Therefore, it offers an enhanced estimation of the electrostatic effect of the protein compared to those obtained previously [27].

Two different trans-axial bases of biological prominence have been considered [35]. The results showed that the DBI ↔ TIm interchange of the trans-axial base has a minor effect on the energy of the Co–C$_R$ bond homolysis. Remarkably, the DFT calculations reveal a minimal but steady increase of the Co–C$_R$ BDE in the Im–[CoIII(corrin)]–R$^+$ model compared to the DBI–[CoIII(corrin)]–R$^+$ model. This indicates that there is a probability of a small steric influence on the axial base of the homolytic dissociation of the Co–C bond. The BDE decreases in the order Me > Rib > Et > ^{i}Prop > ^{t}But and this is in agreement with the variations in the Co–CR bond lengths (Fig. 10.2).

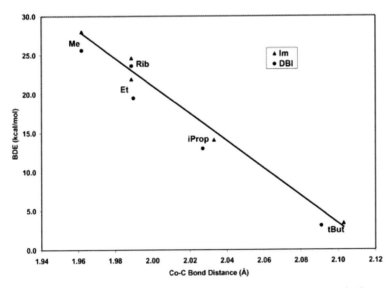

Figure 10.2 Calculated BDEs as a function of the Co–C$_R$ bond lengths [35].

10.4.1 Exercises

1. What atoms in AdoCbl are affected in Co–C bond cleavage?
2. What residues in the protein cause improved Co–C bond cleavage?

3. Why are the reasons for improved Co–C bond cleavage?
4. What interactions are in improved Co–C bond cleavage?

10.5 Structural and Electronic Properties of Vitamin B$_{12}$

Vitamin B$_{12}$, also called Cbls, comprises a central cobalt ion, which is equatorially chelated by a tetradentate corrin macrocycle and is surrounded by two axially coordinating ligands [47]. The lower α-coordinating ligand is a dimethylbenzimidazole (Dmbz) base, which is linked to the f-side chain of the chelator by an α-ribazole containing a backbone [48]. AdoCbl, MeCbl, H$_2$OCbl and CNCbl are examples of Cbls with different β-coordinating ligands [49]. The corrin macrocycle involves four pyrrolic subunits with 14 π-electrons spread over 13 C atoms. The corrin ligand shows prominent differences than the 18 π-electrons containing porphyrins. The boundary of the ligand is completely saturated, and this makes corrinoids structurally flexible with the tight-binding Co ion in different oxidation states. The intensely s-donating property of the macrocycle considerably improves the reactivity of metal-centred Cbl than the Co^{III} complexes. The substitution of axially coordinating ligands was observed to be 10^3 times faster in the Cob(III)alamins complex compared to the Co^{III}–porphyrin complex [50]. This reactivity has also been observed in cofactor B$_{12}$–dependent enzymatic reactions [48]. In the biological structures, Cbl contains square planar Co^I complexes (d^8 electrons), square pyramidal Co^{II} complexes (d^7 electrons) and octahedral Co(III) complexes (d^6 electrons) with distinct coordination geometries. The former comprises a dissociated nucleobase (base-off constitution), as shown in Fig. 10.3.

The base-off forms of Cob(II)alamins and Cob(III)alamins can be achieved by replacing the intramolecular bound Dmbz base with competitive ligands, such as water [51]. This reversible coordination route was aided by the protonation of the Dmbz base. Because the intensity and energy are intensely reliant on the nature of axially coordinating ligands, corrinoids signify a fascinating chromophore for analytical uses [52]. Incomplete corrinoids (i.e. corrinoids lacking the nucleotide base), such as Cob-dicyano-cob(III)yric acid heptamethyl ester, Cob-cyanoaquacob(III)inamide and an intermediate in the biosynthesis of vitamin B_{12} include both artificial B_{12} derivatives and naturally occurring ones. TD-DFT has been used to explore electronically excited states of vitamin B_{12} [8] using the BP86 functional [14, 15] and the 6–31G(d) basis set as applied in Gaussian 03 [53] code. Recent studies showed that the BP86/ 6–31G(d) level of theory was a suitable theoretical parameter for describing the electronic property of vitamin B_{12} [9]. The electronically excited states of vitamin B_{12} have been studied along the elongated Co–CCN bond to check why the Co–C bonds in CNCbl cannot undergo photodissociation under simple photon excitation [8]. The full geometry optimisation was performed for each minimum, and electronic properties related to each optimised structure were analysed. One minimum was defined as excitation having mixed ππ*/metal-to-ligand charge transfer (MLCT) transition, whereas the other was ligand–to–metal charge transfer (LMCT) character. To further comprehend the electronic property of excited states given in Fig. 10.4, frontier orbitals conforming to three different geometries, S_0 minimum (A), the optimised S_1 geometry corresponding to a Co–C bond length of 1.9 Å (B) and the S_1 minimum geometry (C) were obtained from the TD-DFT calculations [7].

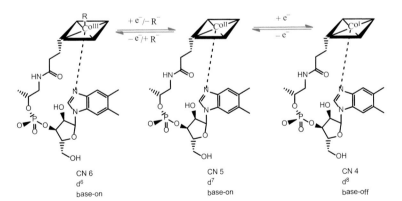

Figure 10.3 Elementary reaction routes for the Co^{III}, Co^{II} and Co^{I} structures of Cbls. CN represents the coordination number [47].

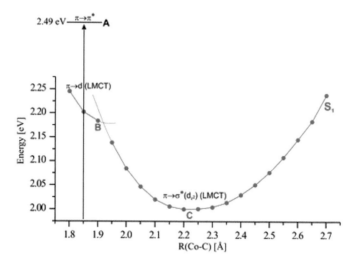

Figure 10.4 Optimised energy of the S_1 state as a function of the Co–C bond length. The energy of the lowest vertical singlet excited states is shown as A and is based on the optimised geometry of the ground states. Point B corresponds to the Co–C bond with a distance of 1.9 Å, while point C corresponds to the S_1 minimum [7].

The HOMO–LUMO excitation was used to determine the lowest singlet excited state of the three geometries. The lowest S_1 excited state is of π–π* character at the S_0 optimised geometry. The character of S_1 state changes to the π–d/p for the same Co–C bond length when its geometry was optimised, and this corresponds to the minimum ground state. Because the antibonding s* orbital has a large influence from the dz² orbital of cobalt, the S_1 state at its optimum geometry can be defined as a LMCT state with elongated axial bonds and was in agreement with earlier experimental studies [11].

References

1. R. J. Sension, D. A. Harris, A. G. Cole, Time-resolved spectroscopic studies of B_{12} coenzymes: comparison of the influence of solvent on the primary photolysis mechanism and geminate recombination of methyl-, ethyl-, n-propyl-, and 5′-deoxyadenosylcobalamin, *J. Phys. Chem. B*, **109** (2005) 21954–21962.
2. T. E. Wiley, W. R. Miller, N. A. Miller, R. J. Sension, P. Lodowski, M. Jaworska, P. M. Kozlowski, Photostability of hydroxocobalamin:

ultrafast excited state dynamics and computational studies, *J. Phys. Chem. Lett.*, **7** (2015) 143–147.

3. A. R. Jones, H. J. Russell, G. M. Greetham, M. Towrie, S. Hay, N. S. Scrutton, Ultrafast infrared spectral fingerprints of vitamin B_{12} and related cobalamins, *J. Phys. Chem. A*, **116** (2012) 5586–5594.

4. J. J. Shiang, A. G. Cole, R. J. Sension, K. Hang, Y. Weng, J. S. Trommel, L. G. Marzilli, T. Lian, Ultrafast excited-state dynamics in vitamin B_{12} and related cob (III) alamins, *J. Am. Chem. Soc.*, **128** (2006) 801–808.

5. A. S. Rury, T. E. Wiley, R. J. Sension, Energy cascades, excited state dynamics, and photochemistry in cob (III) alamins and ferric porphyrins, *Acc. Chem. Res.*, **48** (2015) 860–867.

6. P. M. Kozlowski, B. D. Garabato, P. Lodowski, M. Jaworska, Photolytic properties of cobalamins: a theoretical perspective, *Dalton Trans.*, **45** (2016) 4457–4470.

7. P. Lodowski, M. Jaworska, T. Andruniów, B. D. Garabato, P. M. Kozlowski, Mechanism of the S_1 excited state internal conversion in vitamin B_{12}, *Phys. Chem. Chem. Phys.*, **16** (2014) 18675–18679.

8. P. Lodowski, M. Jaworska, K. Kornobis, T. Andruniów, P. M. Kozlowski, Electronic and structural properties of low-lying excited states of vitamin B_{12}, *J. Phys. Chem. B*, **115** (2011) 13304–13319.

9. K. Kornobis, N. Kumar, B. M. Wong, P. Lodowski, M. Jaworska, T. Andruniów, K. Ruud, P. M. Kozlowski, Electronically excited states of vitamin B_{12}: benchmark calculations including time-dependent density functional theory and correlated *ab initio* methods, *J. Phys. Chem. A*, **115** (2011) 1280–1292.

10. A. Dreuw, M. Head-Gordon, Single-reference *ab initio* methods for the calculation of excited states of large molecules, *Chem. Rev.*, **105** (2005) 4009–4037.

11. D. A. Harris, A. B. Stickrath, E. C. Carroll, R. J. Sension, Influence of environment on the electronic structure of cob (III) alamins: time-resolved absorption studies of the S_1 state spectrum and dynamics, *J. Am. Chem. Soc.*, **129** (2007) 7578–7585.

12. E. Runge, E. K. Gross, Density-functional theory for time-dependent systems, *Phys. Rev. Lett.*, **52** (1984) 997–1000.

13. A. Klamt, G. Schüürmann, COSMO: a new approach to dielectric screening in solvents with explicit expressions for the screening energy and its gradient, *J. Chem. Soc., Perkin Trans. 2*, (1993) 799–805.

14. J. P. Perdew, Density-functional approximation for the correlation energy of the inhomogeneous electron gas, *Phys. Rev. B*, **33** (1986) 8822–8824.

15. A. D. Becke, Density functional thermochemistry III. The role of exact exchange, *J. Chem. Phys.*, **98** (1993) 5648–5652.

16. F. Weigend, M. Häser, H. Patzelt, R. Ahlrichs, RI-MP2: optimized auxiliary basis sets and demonstration of efficiency, *Chem. Phys. Lett.*, **294** (1998) 143–152.

17. O. Treutler, R. Ahlrichs, Efficient molecular numerical integration schemes, *J. Chem. Phys.*, **102** (1995) 346–354.

18. G. N. Schrauzer, G. Parshall, E. Wonchoba, Bis (dimethylglyoximato) cobalt complexes: ("cobaloximes"), *Inorg. Synth.*, **11** (1968) 61–70.

19. K. L. Brown, Chemistry and enzymology of vitamin B_{12}, *Chem. Rev.*, **105** (2005) 2075–2150.

20. L. Randaccio, N. B. Pahor, E. Zangrando, L. Marzilli, Structural properties of organocobalt coenzyme B_{12} models, *Chem. Soc. Rev.*, **18** (1989) 225–250.

21. R. Banerjee, *Chemistry and Biochemistry of B_{12}*, John Wiley & Sons, New York, 1999.

22. M. De March, N. Demitri, S. Geremia, N. Hickey, L. Randaccio, Trans and cis influences and effects in cobalamins and in their simple models, *J. Inorg. Biochem.*, **116** (2012) 215–227.

23. L. Randaccio, S. Geremia, G. Nardin, J. Wuerges, X-ray structural chemistry of cobalamins, *Coord. Chem. Rev.*, **250** (2006) 1332–1350.

24. L. Randaccio, Vitamin B_{12} coenzyme models: perspectives on recent developments in the chemistry of the cobaloximes and related models, *Comments Inorg. Chem.*, **21** (1999) 327–376.

25. L. Randaccio, S. Geremia, E. Zangrando, C. Ebert, Quantitative rationalization of solution and solid state properties in cobaloximes, RCo(DH)2L, as a function of the electronic and steric properties of R, *Inorg. Chem.*, **33** (1994) 4641–4650.

26. J. M. Wood, M. Penley, D. G. Brown, Chemical and biological studies with fluoroalkylcobalamins, *Biochemistry*, **9** (1970) 4302–4310.

27. N. Dölker, F. Maseras, P. E. Siegbahn, Stabilization of the adenosyl radical in coenzyme B_{12}-a theoretical study, *Chem. Phys. Lett.*, **386** (2004) 174–178.

28. P. M. Kozlowski, Quantum chemical modeling of Co–C bond activation in B_{12}-dependent enzymes, *Curr. Opin. Chem. Biol.*, **5** (2001) 736–743.

29. H. M. Marques, K. L. Brown, A molecular mechanics force field for the cobalt corrinoids, *J. Mol. Struct.: THEOCHEM*, **340** (1995) 97–124.

30. H. M. Marques, K. L. Brown, The structure of cobalt corrinoids based on molecular mechanics and NOE-restrained molecular mechanics and dynamics simulations, *Coord. Chem. Rev.*, **190** (1999) 127–153.

31. D. W. Christianson, W. N. Lipscomb, A molecular orbital evaluation of possible factors affecting the homolytic activation of coenzyme B_{12}, *J. Am. Chem. Soc.*, **107** (1985) 2682–2686.

32. L. M. Hansen, P. P. Kumar, D. S. Marynick, Electronic structure of the coenzyme vitamin B_{12} and related systems. 1. $Co(DH)_2(L)$ (R) compounds (DH = dimethylglyoxime; L = NH_3, py, 2-NH2py, 5, 6 dimethylbenzimidazole; R = CH_3, ^{i}-C_3H_7, 5′-deoxyadenosyl) as model systems for the vitamin B_{12} coenzyme, *Inorg. Chem.*, **33** (1994) 728–735.

33. L. Zhu, N. M. Kostic, Molecular orbital study of coenzyme B_{12}. Activation of the cobalt-carbon bond by angular distortions, *Inorg. Chem.*, **26** (1987) 4194–4197.

34. K. P. Jensen, S. P. Sauer, T. Liljefors, P.-O. Norrby, Theoretical investigation of steric and electronic effects in coenzyme B_{12} models, *Organometallics*, **20** (2001) 550–556.

35. P. M. Kozlowski, M. Z. Zgierski, Electronic and steric influence of trans axial base on the stereoelectronic properties of cobalamins, *J. Phys. Chem. B*, **108** (2004) 14163–14170.

36. J. M. Sirovatka, R. G. Finke, Coenzyme B_{12} axial-base chemical precedent studies. Adenosylcobinamide plus sterically hindered axial-base Co–C bond cleavage product and kinetic studies: evidence for the dominance of axial-base transition-state effects and for Co–N (axial-base) distance-dependent, competing σ and π effects, *Inorg. Chem.*, **40** (2001) 1082–1082.

37. J. M. Sirovatka, R. G. Finke, Coenzyme B_{12} axial-base chemical precedent studies. Adenosylcobinamide plus sterically hindered axial-base Co–C bond cleavage product and kinetic studies: evidence for the dominance of axial-base transition-state effects and for Co–N (axial-base) distance-dependent, competing σ and π effects, *Inorg. Chem.*, **38** (1999) 1697–1707.

38. J. M. Sirovatka, A. K. Rappé, R. G. Finke, Molecular mechanics studies of coenzyme B_{12} complexes with constrained Co–N (axial-base) bond lengths: introduction of the universal force field (UFF) to coenzyme B_{12} chemistry and its use to probe the plausibility of an axial-base-

induced, ground-state corrin butterfly conformational steric effect, *Inorg. Chim. Acta*, **300** (2000) 545–555.

39. E. N. G. Marsh, C. L. Drennan, Adenosylcobalamin-dependent isomerases: new insights into structure and mechanism, *Curr. Opin. Chem. Biol.*, **5** (2001) 499–505.

40. F. T. Ng, G. L. Rempel, C. Mancuso, J. Halpern, Decomposition of α-phenethylbis (dimethylglyoximato) cobalt (III) complexes. Influence of electronic and steric factors on the kinetics and thermodynamics of cobalt-carbon bond dissociation, *Organometallics*, **9** (1990) 2762–2772.

41. R. Finke, *In Vitamin B_{12} and B_{12} Proteins*, Wiley-VCH, Weinheim, Germany, 1998.

42. T. Andruniow, M. Z. Zgierski, P. M. Kozlowski, Theoretical determination of the Co–C bond energy dissociation in cobalamins, *J. Am. Chem. Soc.*, **123** (2001) 2679–2680.

43. K. L. Brown, X. Zou, Thermolysis of coenzymes B_{12} at physiological temperatures: activation parameters for cobalt-carbon bond homolysis and a quantitative analysis of the perturbation of the homolysis equilibrium by the ribonucleoside triphosphate reductase from Lactobacillus leichmannii, *J. Inorg. Biochem.*, **77** (1999) 185–195.

44. K. P. Jensen, U. Ryde, Theoretical prediction of the Co–C bond strength in cobalamins, *J. Phys. Chem. A*, **107** (2003) 7539–7545.

45. A. D. Becke, Density-functional exchange-energy approximation with correct asymptotic behavior, *Phys. Rev. A*, **38** (1988) 3098–3100.

46. K. P. Jensen, U. Ryde, How the Co–C bond is cleaved in coenzyme B_{12} enzymes: a theoretical study, *J. Am. Chem. Soc.*, **127** (2005) 9117–9128.

47. F. Zelder, Recent trends in the development of vitamin B_{12} derivatives for medicinal applications, *Chem. Commun.*, **51** (2015) 14004–14017.

48. B. Kräutler, B. T. Golding, D. Arigoni, *Vitamin B_{12} and B_{12}-Proteins*, John Wiley & Sons, New York, 2008.

49. G. Schrauzer, *Inorganic Chemistry of Vitamin B_{12}*, Academic Press, New York, 1972.

50. S. M. Chemaly, M. Florczak, H. Dirr, H. M. Marques, Probing the nature of the Co^{III} ion in corrins: a comparison of the thermodynamics and kinetics of the ligand substitution reactions of aquacyanocobyrinic acid heptamethyl ester and stable yellow aquacyanocobyrinic acid heptamethyl ester, *Inorg. Chem.*, **50** (2011) 8719–8727.

51. K. Zhou, F. Zelder, "Intra base off/inter base on" coordination: self-assembly of a dimeric vitamin B_{12} derivative with a versatile tail, *Chem. Commun.*, **47** (2011) 11999–12001.

52. F. Zelder, L. Tivana, Corrin-based chemosensors for the assured detection of endogenous cyanide, *Org. Biomol. Chem.*, **13** (2015) 14–17.

53. M. Frisch, G. Trucks, H. Schlegel, G. Scuseria, M. Robb, J. Cheeseman, J. Montgomery, T. Vreven, K. Kudin, J. Burant, *Gaussian 03, Revision C.02*, Gaussian, Inc., Wallingford, Connecticut, 2008.

Index

absorption 4, 12, 92
  cellular 121
  electronic 32
acetylcobalamin 104
acid 18, 19, 46
  acetic 130
  amino 4, 44, 117, 123, 125
  carboxylic 18
  cobinic 19
  conjugate 17
  dichlorocobamic 16
  methylmalonic 61
  succinic 53
activation energy 74, 86
adenosylcobalamin (AdoCbl) 9,
    11, 39–41, 44–46, 55, 78,
    80–82, 91, 94, 95, 117, 119,
    120, 122, 124–129, 141, 142,
    149, 150
AdoCbl *see* adenosylcobalamin
adsorption 27, 53, 77
alcohol 12, 25
  allylic 106
  amino 44
  tertiary 104
aldehyde 44, 101–104, 125
alkane 25, 98
alkene 29, 75, 130
  activated 24
  non-activated 24
  prochiral 100, 102
alkylation 24, 27, 47
alkylcobalamin 24, 25, 46, 97, 98,
    107, 127
alkyl halide 24, 25, 27, 91, 97, 98,
    103, 107, 130
  primary 24
  secondary 131

alkyl iodide 25
anaemia 2, 123
animal 1, 60, 61, 64, 80, 92
antidote 44, 52
antivitamins B_{12} 51, 59–62
apoenzyme 78, 142
apoprotein 78
aquacobalamin 17, 22, 27, 51, 70,
    100, 101, 103, 104, 110, 139
aquacorrinoids 52
aquacyanocobalamin 100
aquacyanocobinamide 81
aquahydroxycobinamide 52
aqueous solution 25, 130, 147
aquocobalamin 27
avocado oil 3, 4
aziridines 105, 106

bacteria 1, 60, 124
  methanogenic 92
  nonphotosynthetic 125
BDE *see* bond dissociation energy
benzimidazole 130
benzylalkanes 28
benzyl bromide 108
benzylcobaloxime 28
bicyclic substrate 105, 106
biological process 63, 73, 91, 117
biological system 51, 62, 63, 78
biosynthesis 91, 151
biotin 53, 56
blood 53, 63, 92, 117, 118, 131
blood glucose 52
bond cleavage 82–84, 86, 87, 149,
    150
bond dissociation energy (BDE)
    25, 26, 82–86, 147–149

Index

bond length 31, 84, 85, 141, 142, 146, 151, 152
brain 1, 55, 56, 61, 117, 118
bromodiesters 28
bulk fluid 75, 77

cabamamide 45
cancer 53, 56, 121
  colon 56
  colorectal 56
carbanion 23, 110, 111
carbon 1, 22, 39, 46, 100
  electrophilic 22
  stereogenic 100
carboxymethylcobalamin 131
cardiovascular disease 2, 3, 54, 56
cardiovascular morbidity 55, 57
carotene 4, 125
catalyst 29, 62, 63, 74–77, 80, 81, 87, 94, 103, 104, 107–109, 111, 112
catalytic activity 42, 78, 80–82, 111
catalytic cycle 30, 39, 95, 97, 106, 109, 112
Cbl *see* cobalamin
Cbl derivatives 80, 83, 87, 92, 100, 106, 113
cell 44, 53, 122–124, 131, 132
  diseased 53
  epithelial absorptive 92
  healthy 53
  mammalian 119
  nerve 3, 117
  plant 2
  red blood 1–4, 63, 117
  tumour 56
chemical reaction 43, 74, 80, 130
chemisorption 76
chlorofluorocarbon 75
chloromethyl 110
chloromethylene 110
chlorophenylpropyl 110, 111
chromophore 47, 51, 151

CNCbl *see* cyanocobalamin
cobalamin (Cbl) 16, 17, 22, 41, 42, 45, 51, 60–63, 77, 78, 80–83, 86, 87, 91–93, 98–100, 104, 105, 108–111, 117–119, 125, 126, 128–131, 140, 142, 143, 150, 151
cobaloxime 28, 30, 83
cobalt 4, 9, 16, 21, 40, 46, 47, 78, 104–106, 114, 130, 152
  benign 63
  central 117
  octahedral 42, 122
  triaminomethyl 143
cobamide 16, 17, 19, 22
cobinamide 17–19, 63
cobyrinate 93, 100
coenzymes 39–41, 43, 44, 46, 47, 78, 81, 82, 85, 86, 95, 118, 119, 122, 141, 143
  acetyl 92
  bioactive 124
cofactor 21, 61, 63, 64, 78, 81, 117, 119, 122, 124, 125, 139, 142
cognitive function 2, 57, 58
conditions
  aerobic 25, 125
  anaerobic 25, 44, 127
  electrochemical 103
  medical 2
  neurological 55
  oxygen-free 130
  reaction 29, 105, 108
conductor-like screening model 141
corrin 9–11, 27, 45, 46, 83–86, 141, 143–149
corrin macrocycle 100, 150
corrinoids 11, 16, 21, 22, 51, 52, 61, 150, 151
coupling reaction 77, 93, 106, 108
cyanide 27, 45, 46, 51, 52, 118, 121
cyanide detection 51, 52, 63

cyanide detoxification 51, 52, 118, 121
cyanide poisoning 44, 45, 121
cyanocobalamin (CNCbl) 1, 17, 27, 41, 44–46, 78, 80, 81, 99–102, 105–109, 117, 119–122, 129–131, 140, 141, 150, 151
cyclisation 25, 103, 109, 111
cyclohexenone 103
cyclohexylcobalamin 78, 131
cyclopropanation 77, 93, 109
cyclopropane 105, 106, 109, 111

dairy products 1, 119
dehalogenation 63, 77, 91, 93, 97, 114
    catalysed 81
    reductive 78
dementia 2, 56
density functional theory (DFT) 31, 141–143, 149
deoxyadenosine 9, 27
deoxyadenosylcobalamin 25, 45
detoxification 51, 52, 63, 73, 118
DFT *see* density functional theory
diabetes 3, 53, 54
diabetic neuropathy 122, 123
diarrhoea 3, 130
diffusion 76, 77
disease 3, 123, 132
    Alzheimer's 3, 119
    degenerative 60
    heart 3, 54, 58
    inflammatory bowel 3
    Leber's 4
    liver 130
    nerve 61
    renal 57
disorder 45, 53, 55, 92
    mental 3
    nerve 123
    nervous 119
    neuropsychiatric 2
    sleep 3, 121

DNA 4, 45, 61, 111, 112, 117, 118, 125, 131
DNA synthesis 1, 55, 63, 73, 91, 93
drug 53, 56, 73
    anticancer 56
    antiproliferative 59
    antivitamin-based 59
    peptide/protein 54

electrolysis 27, 30, 103, 109, 110
electron paramagnetic resonance (EPR) 44, 53
electron-withdrawing group (EWG) 103–106
enthalpy 26
enzymatic process 21, 26, 60, 91
enzymatic reaction 4, 63, 78, 81, 150
enzyme 39–46, 61–64, 73, 78, 81–83, 85, 86, 92, 94, 114, 117, 119, 122–127, 147, 148
    mammalian 42
epilepsy 55, 56
EPR *see* electron paramagnetic resonance
Escherichia coli 23, 43, 61
ester 29, 30, 75, 103, 104, 151
ethanol 12, 96
EWG *see* electron-withdrawing group

FA *see* folic acid
folic acid (FA) 4, 53, 54, 56–58, 117, 123

gastrectomy 60
gastrointestinal tract 54
glycerol 93, 127, 128

halocobalamin 97, 98
heterolysis 91, 95, 96, 102, 127, 143
histidine 85, 129

Index

homocysteine 2, 41, 42, 54, 58, 61, 92, 120, 122, 123
homolysis 25, 30, 82, 85, 91, 94, 98, 107, 108, 110, 112, 113, 143, 144, 147
homolytic cleavage 26, 29, 78, 82, 106–108, 110, 125, 132, 143, 147
homolytic fission 127, 128
hydrogenation 75, 93, 100, 103, 104
hydroxocobalamin 16, 17, 22, 24, 44, 45, 47, 55, 112, 117, 119, 120, 128, 131

insulin 53, 54
isomerisation 63, 78, 91, 94, 114
itching 4, 130

Leber's hereditary optic atrophy 44
ligand 10, 16, 26, 53, 81–85, 141–143, 150
  α-coordinating 150
  active-site 30
  alpha axial 84, 85
  β-coordinating 41, 150
  beta 79, 83, 84
  beta aqua 112
  cis 83
  corrin 11, 21, 26, 150
  donor 87
  high-affinity 61
  histidine 40
  molecular 53
  strong field 27
  trans 83
liver 1, 52, 54, 80, 125

macrocycle 52, 85, 150
  corrole 85
  nickel-containing 43
magnetic circular dichroism (MCD) 32, 126

mammal 59–63, 73, 80, 124
MCD see magnetic circular dichroism
MCM see methylmalonyl-CoA mutase
MeCbl see methylcobalamin
mechanism 9, 42, 98, 106, 111, 127, 139, 141–143
  analgesic 123
  cob-independent 42
  enzymatic 141
  homolytic 29
  microscopic 125
  molecular 31
  pathophysiological 55
  photostability 140
  radical 29
  reductive 111
metabolism 4, 12, 41, 55, 57, 60, 64, 73, 92, 124
methane 43, 92
methanogenesis 43, 92
methionine 42, 61, 92, 120, 122, 123, 125
methionine synthase 21, 39–43, 64, 92, 95, 122
methyl cation 82, 91, 95, 96, 99
methylcobalamin (MeCbl) 9, 11, 21, 22, 24, 31, 39–45, 63, 64, 78, 80–82, 91, 95–97, 99, 100, 117, 119–124, 141, 142
methyl group 4, 9, 16, 24, 39, 42, 43, 64, 78, 81, 84, 95–97
methylmalonyl-CoA mutase (MCM) 39–41, 45, 64, 93, 119, 124
methyltransferases 31, 39, 42, 43, 63, 92
microorganism 1, 42, 64, 92, 131

nerve 118, 123
  injured 124
  optical 4
  sciatic 124

wounded 124
neurons 119, 124
NMR *see* nuclear magnetic resonance
nuclear magnetic resonance (NMR) 11, 127
nucleophiles 23, 95, 105

orbital 143, 152
organic reaction 77, 87, 113, 114
organocobalamin 29
organylcobalamin 25
oxidation 25, 43, 47, 75, 78, 93, 111
oxidation state 16, 47, 78, 82, 125, 150

pathway 29, 42, 128
  methionine salvage 41
  translocation 21
patient 2, 53–55, 57–59, 123
  diabetics 123
  renal 54
pernicious anaemia 2, 3, 41, 55, 92, 122, 130
PES *see* potential energy surface
pesticide 81
photolysis 104, 125, 127, 129, 131, 132, 139
Ping-Pong reaction 42
porphyrins 4, 9–11, 85, 150
potential energy surface (PES) 140, 141
protein 2, 12, 40, 42, 43, 53, 57, 64, 92, 125–127, 129, 148, 149
psoriasis 3, 4
pyridoxine 58
pyrroles 9

radiationless deactivation 140, 141
randomised controlled trial (RCT) 54, 56–58

RCT *see* randomised controlled trial
reactant 75, 104
reaction 24, 25, 39, 40, 42, 43, 63, 74, 77, 80–82, 100–104, 108, 111, 113, 147
  allergic 130
  amidation 53
  deamination 93
  dehalogenation 63
  enzyme-catalysed 141
  oxidisation 46
  radical 64, 132
  ring expansion 29, 30, 113
  ring-opening 93, 105
reactivity 22, 30, 39, 51, 64, 80, 150
reduction 27, 43, 47, 58, 73, 75, 82, 86, 93, 97, 101, 102, 130
  enzymatic 44
  nitrile 100
  one-electron 27
ribonucleotides 93
ring expansion 29, 30, 77, 93

saturated calomel electrode 27
seizures 55
smoke inhalation 44, 45
smoke poisoning 132
species 30–32
  active carbon 105
  active Co-aqua 112
  nucleophilic 130
species-associated difference spectra 139
steric effect 84, 85, 142, 143, 145
steric hindrance 84, 130
styrene 107–110
styrene derivatives 28, 29, 108
substrate 21, 29, 30, 39, 43, 80, 81, 94–96, 100, 102, 105, 126
synthesis 4, 25, 27, 55, 92, 113, 117, 123, 130

chemical 63
melatonin 121, 123
myelin 123
organic 29, 63, 113

TD-DFT *see* time-domain density functional theory
time-domain density functional theory (TD-DFT) 139–141, 151
titanium 99, 100
tobacco amblyopia 44
transmethylation 77, 95, 97, 114

urine 45, 121

vacuum 86, 148
vanadium trichloride 113
van der Waals interactions 86
vasodilation 45
vinylcobalamin 22, 131
vitamin 4, 9, 47, 53, 55–60, 64, 78, 79, 91, 108, 117, 118
vitamin B_{12} 1–4, 9–12, 15 17, 21, 22, 27, 28, 44–47, 51–57, 60, 61, 63, 64, 77–82, 91, 92, 96–98, 102–106, 110–112, 117, 119–124, 129–132, 139–143, 147, 150, 151
vitamin B_{12} deficiency 2, 3, 55, 60–62, 119, 121, 122